P9-ASJ-068

MANAGING STRESS

A businessperson's guide by
JERE E. YATES

MANAGING STRESS

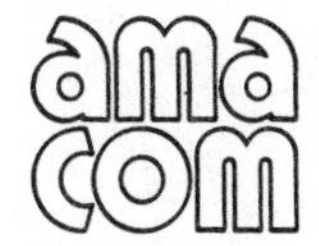

a division of American Management Associations

Library of Congress Cataloging in Publication Data

Yates, Jere E
Managing stress.

Bibliography: p.
Includes index.
1. Job stress. 2. Executives—Psychology.
I. Title.
HF5548.85.Y37 158.7 79-15564
ISBN 0-8144-5543-3

First Printing

To Carolyn, Camille, Kevin,
and Brian, with whom I have
experienced the whole range of
stress, from the agony of distress
to the thrill of eustress.

PREFACE

Stress is one of the most used yet least understood words in the English language. Most people assume that stress is bad for you. This is not always the case: Stress in proper amounts is a necessary ingredient in any person whose life is going to manifest vitality. Stress is to be *managed,* not simply avoided.

Stress management is important for everyone. This book specifically addresses the manager's concern with effectively managing his own stress as well as that of the people under his supervision, although, anyone could read and profit from the book. For example, a manager's spouse could read the book and gain from it personally as well as be able to better help his or her partner.

Few tasks that face managers are more important than stress management, because excessive levels of stress over a prolonged period of time can lead to physical, psychological, or emotional distress. This distress is very damaging to the individual's health and very costly to an organization in terms of loss in productivity and increased disability and insurance premiums. This book is written to show managers how—by managing stress in themselves and in the people they supervise—they can contribute to the prevention of illness while improving productivity and reducing costs.

I am indebted to the following persons who have contributed to this book: Ruth D. Atteberry, whose editorial assistance was superb;

Pepperdine University's Seaver College, which provided clerical support; Earl Ends, whose speech on stress first prompted my interest in the topic; Robert G. Wright, who gave direction and encouragement; Walter R. Berg and Hughes Aircraft Company, where I developed some of my ideas while doing stress management workshops; and my family for their emotional and spiritual support.

Jere E. Yates

CONTENTS

INTRODUCTION

The Costs of Stress to Business

According to the U.S. Clearinghouse for Mental Health Information, during the last few years U.S. industry has suffered a $17 billion annual decrease in productivity losses as a result of stress-related mental disorders. Estimates on productivity losses as a result of stress-related physical illnesses are even higher—$60 billion! And illnesses caused by stress have resulted in significant losses in wages to workers ($8.6 billion lost annually to cardiovascular diseases alone, many of which are thought to be associated with high levels of stress).

Stress-related accidents and disabilities are becoming a major cost for both the public and private sectors. According to the *Los Angeles Times,* $1.8 billion was paid in 1976 by employers in California to maintain a workers' compensation system that paid over $1.2 billion in benefits to approximately 1 million workers injured or killed on their jobs.[1] Across the country the total premium costs were well over $8 billion. In the past five years the costs of disability pensions in the County of Los Angeles has tripled. Stress disability claims are driving up costs in every organization, whether it is self-insured or is covered by a state workers' compensation system. It's an indication of how serious a medical problem stress is for the American people and how costly this problem can be from an economic perspective.

Yet economic costs hardly reflect all the human costs involved as a result of illness. These costs include emotional traumas associated with illness and reduced income, as well as the personal suffering that comes from stress-related drug addiction and alcoholism. Much of this human suffering can't be measured financially, but its impact is nonetheless damaging to individuals.

These costs of stress to business are prompting many companies to fight back to reduce both financial and human costs by encouraging their employees to manage stress more effectively. Preventative health programs designed to reduce stress and improve overall health, such as the one at Kimberly-Clark Corporation, are springing up all over the country, and for good reason: In 1977 insurance premiums for 15,000 employees cost Kimberly-Clark $14.3 million, 75 percent more than they did in 1973!

Stress management programs are a real bargain. They cost relatively little and they can conceivably save millions of dollars a year in this country alone. This book can be profitably used by individuals and organizations alike to reduce the amount of human suffering and economic loss that has been caused by stress-related diseases.

REFERENCE

1. *Los Angeles Times,* June 18, 1977.

CHAPTER 1

Stress and the Life of a Modern Manager

Chronic stress is the major health problem facing managers in America today. We live in an age where we have almost completely eliminated many infectious diseases that historically have wiped out entire civilizations. (Children in America are no longer vaccinated for smallpox because the risk associated with immunization is greater than the likelihood of catching the disease!) But we are being victimized by stress, an insidious form of illness which comes as a result of our prosperity and of the pace at which we live in this technologically sophisticated world. A Tulsa reporter, Judy Randle, put it well:

> . . . In a society where 60 percent of the visits to a doctor are for signs of distress rather than a specific illness, where the top ten causes of death include only one infectious disease, and where the most highly prescribed drugs are tranquilizers, people need to be aware of stress and its effects.[1]

We are indeed victims of our own technology! None of us wants to give up the most luxurious style of living that man has ever known, nor do we want to turn back the clock and give up modern conveniences such as fast planes and cars that whisk us to our destinations in minutes or hours. Yet the speed of our modern machines has caused our own internal systems to speed up, moving at an ever faster pace, and creating what some are now calling the "hurry sickness."

Stress-related diseases are real. They do cause people to get sick—

they can even kill. Excessive stress has been linked to many different kinds of illness from low-back pain to cancer. In this chapter I shall highlight what is known about the relationship of stress to these various diseases and focus on the kind of turbulent, changing world in which the manager works, lives, and plays.

Stress and the heart

Nearly one million Americans die each year from cardiovascular disease, accounting for almost 55 percent of all deaths. In recent years almost 700,000 Americans have died annually of heart attacks, one third of these deaths among people under the age of 65. The National Heart, Lung, and Blood Institute recently estimated that 1.3 million Americans would experience coronary disease. Interestingly, heart disease became a major health problem only at the beginning of this century. Between 1940 and 1950 the rate of coronary artery disease for white males aged 35 to 64 increased by 23 percent. Although very recently there has been a slight decline in mortality due to coronary disease, this trend is hardly encouraging—coronary disease is still the major cause of death in America. The average American male has a one-in-five chance of having a heart attack before he reaches the age of 60, and those who live the hard-charging, competitive, aggressive style favored by corporations will have an even greater likelihood of succumbing to heart disease.

Despite all the public interest in cardiovascular disease as the number one killer in this country, we have only recently begun to recognize the relationship between this disease and stress. Such factors as high levels of cholesterol and of fatty substances, hypertension (high blood pressure), obesity, heredity, an inactive life style, a diabetic condition, and heavy cigarette smoking have long been associated with cardiovascular illness. The work of such men as Dr. Meyer Friedman, a San Francisco cardiologist, and Dr. Hans Selye, a medical researcher whose stress institute at the University of Montreal is probably the best known in the world, has provided considerable evidence of a direct relationship between stress and heart disease.

Dr. Selye contends that the above-mentioned factors associated with heart disease cause only the *preconditions* for a heart attack; they do not by themselves actually bring on an attack. He believes that the decisive, eliciting factor is excessive stress. But this is more than just a mere belief; Dr. Selye has demonstrated in his laboratory that heart accidents can be induced chemically by excessive stress, even without occlusion (closing) of arteries in the heart![2]

Physicians have long known that heart attacks occur primarily among what has been called "coronary candidates," people who— in addition to the above-mentioned predisposing factors—have an aggressive, overactive personality. Dr. Selye took some purebred rats and gave them a combination of hormones and sodium salt, which caused no visible cardiac damage but did turn them into "coronary candidates." Forced exercise, frustration—almost any kind of stressor brought on death caused by cardiac failure. There is also evidence that acute emotional stress may bring on sudden death by unalterably interrupting the rhythm of the heart even though no actual tissue dies. Selye cites the work of Dr. George L. Engel of Rochester, New York, who has taken numerous case reports on sudden death due to psychological stress and has put them in the following eight categories: (1) on the impact of death of a close friend or relative; (2) during severe grief; (3) at the threat of losing a close friend or relative; (4) during mourning or on an anniversary; (5) on the loss of self-esteem or of status; (6) when faced with personal danger or the threat of injury; (7) after the danger has passed; and (8) during a reunion, triumph, or happy ending.

Drs. Friedman and Rosenman also have made a great contribution to our knowledge of the relationship between heart disease and a certain personality or behavior pattern, which they call Type A behavior. The person with a Type A personality is two to three times more likely to suffer from coronary artery disease than the person who has the opposite characteristics—the Type B personality. Type A people have a chronic, incessant struggle with time, always trying to get the most done in the least amount of time; they are very competitive and aggressive; and they usually have a hostility that lies just below the surface and is easily provoked. Type B people have some of these same qualities, but not in as chronic or pronounced a form as do Type A personalities.

Stress and hypertension

Between 23 and 44 million Americans are currently suffering from hypertension (high blood pressure), and almost half of these people don't even know they have it. Hypertension is the major contributing factor to heart disease and is responsible by itself for some 60,000 deaths a year. To state it a bit more bluntly: If you are hypertensive, you are four times as likely to have a heart attack or a stroke as is someone with normal blood pressure, and twice as likely to develop kidney disease, which accounts for 60,000 deaths a year. According to actuarial tables, a 35-year-old man who has a blood pressure reading of 150/100 will have a life expectancy of 16½ fewer years than his counterpart with a reading of 120/80. A 45-year-old man with the higher reading would have 11½ fewer years than his counterpart; for the 55-year-old man, the difference would be six fewer years. The conclusion is obvious: At any age, the higher one's blood pressure, the shorter will be one's life expectancy. But this situation is by no means irredeemable—hypertension can be treated with drugs, diet, and changes in life style. As a leading researcher, Dr. John Henry Laragh of New York's Columbia Presbyterian Medical Center, has said: "Hypertension does not have to be the single leading factor in disability and death in the U.S. today. We have the means to control it."[3]

As blood is driven through the body's circulatory system by the heart's pumping action, pressure is exerted on the walls of the various blood vessels. Although necessary to transport oxygen-carrying blood to all parts of the body, this pressure must be carefully controlled by some rather complex mechanisms. Baroceptors signal the nervous system to lower or raise pressure by contracting or dilating arterioles or by slowing down or speeding up the heart beat. Arteries can tolerate high blood pressure only for brief surges, and vessels can't tolerate high pressure any more than pipes can tolerate high water pressure for prolonged periods. Normal functioning does allow for a rise in blood pressure during exercise or excitement and a fall in blood pressure during periods of sleep or relaxation.

High blood pressure is particularly hazardous to the brain and heart. It can create a blowout or rupture of an artery that supplies the brain with oxygen, thus precipitating a stroke because some part of the brain was denied the oxygen it so desperately needed. High blood pressure can also adversely affect the heart itself: Because the heart must pump against increased resistance, high blood pressure forces the heart to work much harder than it usually does. This additional work creates the need for more oxygen than the system can provide, perhaps bringing on the familiar chest pains of angina pectoris or even some irreplaceable damage to the heart muscle. Or, as a result of overworking, the enlarged heart may not be able to empty itself against the pressure of blood in the arteries, thus causing fluid to build up behind the heart, lungs, and extremities and bringing on the heart attack.

Even though hypertension can be treated, we are still uncertain about its cause. Such factors as obesity, heredity, diet, race, and stress are strongly suspected as culprits. For every extra pound on your body, there is a corresponding increase in blood volume, which causes the heart to work harder to pump the blood to each each extra pound of fatty tissue. If your family has a history of hypertension, you are statistically in a higher risk group than someone whose family does not have such a history.

Diet has been linked to hypertension as we have come to better grasp the impact of salt on the system. According to Dr. Laragh, "Salt is the hydraulic agent of life. It is salt that holds the water in humans, causes swelling and a high fluid volume. This means an increased blood pressure." Race may also be a factor in hypertension, because one of every four adult black Americans has high blood pressure, whereas only one of seven adult whites has it. It may be related to a genetically transmitted incapacity to handle large amounts of salt in highly seasoned "soul food," or simply due to the pressures of being black in a predominately white society. William Grier and Price Cobb, two black psychiatrists, have said that the high incidence of hypertension among blacks comes from "being black, and perpetually angry, and unable to express it or do anything about it."[4]

Stress also has been identified as a cause of hypertension. Although there is some question about just how much of a factor it is in the origin of the illness, there is no question about the unfavorable effects stress may have on an existing hypertensive condition.[5] When the body encounters real or imagined threats, it responds instantly by increasing the blood pressure in order to rush an oversupply of blood to vital parts of the body. When the threat has subsided, the blood pressure ordinarily drops back down to normal levels, but not if the body is still faced with anxiety, fear, or hostility. If some unconscious threat remains, the pressure may remain high, creating unnecessary, long-term stress on the complex network of blood vessels. Even when the threat has completely disappeared, the pressure may not drop all the way back to normal: Each time this reaction occurs, the pressure may drop by smaller amounts, eventually stabilizing at a permanently high level. One study indicated that men who had lost their jobs experienced increases in blood pressure that persisted until they found new jobs. Even though the relationship between stress and hypertension may not be quite as strong as that between stress and heart disease, there is a relationship. Stress also has been linked to many other ailments that plague us.

Stress and cancer

Cancer claims the lives of approximately 750,000 Americans each year. Some researchers believe that it is related to excessive stress. Dr. Eugene P. Pendergrass, a former president of the American Cancer Society, has observed that many patients seem to have their cancers reactivated, after apparently successful treatment, by the onset of some acute form of stress such as the death of a son or the end of long-term employment,[6] and in many cases this recurrence proves fatal.

Lawrence Leshan of New York's Institute of Applied Biology studied 450 cancer patients for 12 years. He discovered that these cancer patients had three psychological characteristics in common more frequently than a control group of people not suffering from cancer.[7] First, the majority of them had experienced the loss of a very important personal relationship before their disease was identified (and presumably before its onset). Second, almost half of them displayed an inability to vent hostile feelings toward others. Third, more than one third of them displayed a manifest level of tension concerning the death of one of their parents even when the death had occurred some time back.

The social-stress theory of cancer is not as yet widely supported by scientific research, but it is receiving increasing attention. For instance, Dr. W. B. Gross, a professor of veterinary medicine at Virginia Polytechnic Institute, discovered that chickens whose pecking order was disrupted by researchers (an example of social stress) were eight times as likely to get cancer as a group of chickens whose pecking order remained intact.[4]

Dr. Jack E. White, director of the cancer research center at Howard University Medical School, has reported that between 1950 and 1967 the mortality rate for all types of cancer among black males jumped 50 percent.[4] The combined rate for black males and females increased 20 percent, while the rate among whites showed no comparable increase. Although Dr. White attributes this increase to environmental factors such as more exposure to pollutants in the air in the city than on the farm, he does believe that stress may be an important factor as well.

We know very little about the possible relationship between stress and cancer. Yet we do know enough to justify much more research. This research is especially warranted when one realizes that investigators are reporting with increasing regularity that stress is associated with increased susceptibility to illness in general.

Stress and other illnesses

The causal relationship between stress and physical illness is a most amazing phenomenon indeed. Ritual executions through the practice of voodoo are examples of how powerful an effect extreme stress can have upon an individual, especially when social support is withdrawn, because a person is then seen by friends as being as good as dead. Walter Cannon, the noted Harvard physiologist, discovered that the practice of voodoo subjects a person's nervous system to intolerable loads of stress.[6] The heart develops arrhythmia because it's exhausted by overstimulation—it quivers but does not pulse or beat. It is a self-fulfilling prophecy: Believing that death is imminent, the person waits in fear or resignation until he or she does die.

Although such an extreme response to stress is real, most American managers will not encounter witch doctors practicing voodoo in corporate life! (At least they will not be easily recognized as such: Some would claim that corporate voodoo of sorts does exist!) But we do face a multitude of physical illnesses that have been tied directly to excessive stress loads. Although most researchers agree that stress brings on an increased generalized susceptibility to illness, others have not been able to corroborate any direct relationship between stress and specific diseases. Selye has rather clearly indicated in his work that whereas some diseases have specific causes (a particular germ or poison), others result more from the body's own excessive reaction to some unusual situation.[2] This overreaction has prompted Selye to speak of these stress-related diseases as "diseases of adaptation" because they are actually caused by the body's maladaptation. It seems that health exists when the mind and body are functioning in harmony, and illness besets us when stress upsets this harmony and balance.

STRESS AND ULCERS

The connection between stress and ulcers has always been strong in the public's mind. It is estimated that 5 percent of the American population suffers periodically from ulcers, but these statistics show that ulcers are no laughing matter—particularly if you have one. Incredibly, some people are *proud* of their ulcers, because they are seen as "purple hearts" for living a productive life.

It is common knowledge that gastric and duodenal ulcers occur far more often in people who are always tense over family and work problems than in those who aren't. Constant stress keeps the gastric system working full time, whether it is necessary or not. Bleeding ulcers can be brought on overnight by intense stress levels. People who suffered severe burns and people who lived through air raids during the war have been found to react to extreme emotional excitement in this way. Ulcerative colitis, a disease of the colon characterized by bleeding ulcerations, is another serious form ulcers take, and it can be fatal. Diet may be related to ulcers as well, but as Dr. I. Mendeloff, former president of the American Gastroenterological Association, put it: "It's what's eating you rather than what you're eating" that is the real culprit in the development of ulcers.[4]

STRESS AND DIABETES

Although a predisposition to diabetes is certainly inherited, it is also true that whether a latent diabetic tendency develops into the full-blown disease depends largely upon the way the body reacts to stress.

Normally the blood sugar level is raised when a person is under stress. When the condition is prolonged, an excessive burden is placed upon the pancreas so that it finally fails in its efforts to produce enough insulin, the hormone that enables glucose to penetrate individual cells and to create actual energy. There is plenty of evidence connecting diabetes with stress and demonstrating that a diabetic's condition worsens under stress.[7]

BACKACHES AND HEADACHES

Backaches and headaches are two common results of excessive stress. For example, headaches cause more than half the visits to physicians' offices, and migraine headaches will strike one in eight Americans at some point in their lives. The migraine headache is distinct from the muscular tension headache. The migraine is caused by dilation of the blood vessels in the head. Harold G. Wolff has pointed out a paradoxical fact about stress and migraines: People tend to get migraines not when stress is at its peak, but shortly after the pressure has lifted. Sunday, for example, is a popular day for getting migraine headaches, because Sunday is "the day of rest" after the hectic work week.

Most cases of back pain are caused by muscular tension or weakness. Our sedentary habits contribute to weak back muscles, and the hectic pace of life today—with all its pressures—can cause tension which is frequently concentrated in the region of the lower back. Prolonged tightening of these muscles can induce pain.

STRESS AND ALLERGIES

It's common knowledge that people get sick when they are run down. What's not as well known is that people also get sick when their resistance is too high. Allergies result when the "body is injured . . . by its own protective devices, senselessly firing away at harmless challenge, sometimes at no challenge at all."[7] When people are exposed to something to which they are allergic, their bodies overreact and release chemicals, such as histamine, in quantities that make the impact of the body's defensive reaction far worse than the disease itself. This condition is essentially a breakdown in the body's immunological system. Many allergists believe that emotional problems can precipitate allergic attacks, as well as exacerbate existing allergic conditions. Interestingly, in some cases the body can respond hypersensitively even to a picture of the irritant. For example, some people who are allergic to hay may have an allergic reaction when they are shown a picture of haystacks!

Asthma is the most common allergic disease in developed countries, and is thought to afflict 5 percent of the people. Its greater prevalence in developed than in underdeveloped countries may be caused in part by the stress associated with a more industrialized life style. Particularly among young asthmatics, one can see the effects of emotional excitement. One five-year-old boy was so severely developmentally disabled that his parents placed him in a facility that could provide 24-hour care and therapy, although they regularly took him home to spend the night. The child was asthmatic, and before long a pattern began to emerge: Every time he was brought back to the facility after staying overnight with his parents, the child would have an asthma attack, but if he was not kept overnight, he normally did not have an attack. The explanation appeared to be that when the child was home for prolonged periods, he became emotionally very excited, thus precipitating the asthma attack.

STRESS AND ARTHRITIS

Although the causes of rheumatoid arthritis are not clearly understood, stress has been demonstrated to be positively correlated with arthritis.[8] As the chief cause of physical disability among Americans, arthritis affects approximately 50 million people, and about 17 million of these cases are severe enough to require ongoing medical attention. Apparently a breakdown in the immunological system occurs, and this breakdown may be caused by stress. The malfunctioning of the immunological system has the following effect: As antibodies fight an infection in the joints, they fail to distinguish between healthy and unhealthy cells. The result is a painful inflammation of the joints which in mild cases is only irritating but in severe cases can confine people to wheelchairs or beds.

STRESS AND SEXUAL DYSFUNCTIONS

Although all sexual dysfunctions are not caused by stress, excessive stress is responsible at times for impotence and premature ejaculation in men and for frigidity in women. Besides decreasing sexual desire in men, stress also inhibits the formation of sperm cells. The sexual prowess of a man is linked directly to his production of the male hormone testosterone, and Dr. Robert Rose of the Boston University School of Medicine has demonstrated that as stress goes up, testosterone goes down.[4] In women, stress can cause insufficient milk supply during lactation, or even the total cessation of milk production for awhile. Of course, in men and women sexual dysfunctions or irregularities are quite likely to create even greater stress the more people fret about the problem. Because we live in a society that constantly pushes the idea of adequacy in sexual performance, minor sexual dysfunctions induced by a temporary stress situation are blown out of proportion and become major sexual and psychological problems. (In Chapter 5, I shall demonstrate how a healthy sex life can be a real asset in dealing with stress successfully.)

Stress and change

In his historic book, *Future Shock,* Alvin Toffler depicted our changing, turbulent world in which we are faced with so much change, so much information to absorb, and so many decisions and choices to make, that we frequently end up in a disoriented and confused state because of our inability to cope adequately with such a vast amount of change.[9] Toffler suggests that change will be continuous and that its pace will even accelerate in the future. A few years ago John Gardner said that the only kind of stability we have today is "stability in motion"[10] Things that appear to be stable just *appear* to be stable; they may just be changing less rapidly.

Most of us fail to recognize the degree to which change has occurred in our own generation. Toffler provides somewhat of a historical perspective by indicating that if you take the last 50,000 years of man's existence and divide it into lifetimes of 62 years each, you will end up with approximately 800 lifetimes, 650 of which were spent in caves. Writing was invented only 70 lifetimes ago; printing, only six lifetimes ago. Only during the last four lifetimes has it been possible to measure time with any accuracy, and the electric motor has been here for just the last two lifetimes. In fact, most of the material goods to which we are accustomed were invented in the current lifetime, number 800. The computer has a pervasive influence in the world today, yet Univac I came out only in 1954. We have therefore seen a total computer revolution in just 25 years. Who knows what new inventions will have a similar revolutionary impact on our lives? One thing that we do know is that the rate of change in all areas of society shows no sign of slackening in the immediate future.

Stress and women

Nowhere is the effect of rapid change more apparent than in the changing role of today's woman, who is subjected to pressure from all sides. If she does pursue a career in addition to rearing a family, she must be adept at balancing her business and personal affairs in order to have enough time for all her demands. Unless she is blessed with a "liberated" husband, she may still be doing a disproportionate share of housework—washing, ironing, cleaning, and cooking—so that in effect, her job is piled on top of her many household responsibilities. As a result she lives at a frenzied pace, with little time for personal or social involvements.

Women also face severe tests at work. Many women believe that to gain recognition on the job they have to be 100 percent better than a man is. Whether true or not (and it probably is), this perception of the situation can cause a woman to drive herself more than is healthy for her. A strong, assertive woman is accused of being pushy; a weaker, less assertive woman is criticized for not being tough enough to survive in a dog-eat-dog world, so she feels damned if she does and damned if she doesn't. A woman manager also has to deal with the discomfort that many men and women feel about this reversal of traditional roles.

A woman may also be driving herself much too hard at home to prove to her family that her professional work isn't going to interfere with her traditional roles of wife and mother. The end result may be disastrous for "super-mom" because the pace is too intense and too unreal for anyone.

Then there is the woman who is trying to "go it alone." Perhaps she has a family, but is recently divorced and is now going to work for the first time. She may resent having given so many years to her husband and children and, as a result, not having the education or experience to get a job that pays well. Yet her pride pushes her on: She is determined to prove to herself and to everyone else that she can make it on her own. Financial pressures are usually high, because she must get some help around the house or with young children. Without a spouse to help her with household chores and to provide emotional support, she often feels pulled in many directions and taxed beyond her resources. She may find it difficult to give her children all they need, because she is worn out at the end of the day; yet she must still cook, wash, clean, and help her children with their homework. It is no wonder that she is often depressed, impatient, short of temper, and completely fatigued.

It is also interesting to see the effect of the women's liberation movement on those married women who are only working at home. The housewife of today frequently questions the honorableness of her "work." She may feel guilty that she is not pursuing a career, since all the attention appears to be going to those women who are in the business world. She may also worry about how she will be able to work productively after her children have grown and have left the house. She may experience feelings of doubt, inferiority, and anxiety as she faces an uncertain future for which she is ill prepared, and both she and her friends may question the validity of her position. The cumulative effect of these worries is stressful.

These pressures on women at work and at home are bound to take their toll: Stress-ridden people do tend to get ill more frequently than others. As you might expect, just within the past decade there has been a perceptible increase in deaths from heart disease among women. We don't know exactly how to account for this rise, but researchers are strongly suspicious of the impact of new cultural values and expectations that have emerged from the movement to liberate women from their traditional roles. This social change is probably much harder on women than on men, and women who choose to remain at home are sometimes subject to as much pressure as those who enter the world of men's work.

Here is an illustration of this new, unexpected vulnerability of women to stress-related illness. A 33-year-old woman who had a very responsible position with a major government agency invited me to present a one-day workshop for her people on how to manage stress more effectively in their lives. She said, "My staff just doesn't seem to be coping very well with the pressures of living. They seem to be harried, confused, upset, irritable, impatient, and full of tension—not only occasionally, but all the time." So I agreed to present a stress management workshop for her and her people. As it turned out, the day I was there doing the workshop, this young woman "had" to be in Washington. One week later she had a heart attack! Now I'm not presumptuous enough to say that if she had attended my session, she wouldn't have had the attack. What I am suggesting is that she, like many other young women, was under the delusion that she of all people was not likely to suffer from heart disease—after all, she was a *young* woman!

Managerial implications

Given this kind of world, there seem to be two major implications for managers. One is that we had better develop the right attitude toward change. A willingness to accept any and every change is no more workable an attitude for the manager today than is resistance to every change. We must be discriminating in our selection of the kinds of changes we want to bring about in our lives. As managers we need to be *proactive* rather than *reactive,* anticipating the kinds of changes we desire to make and trying to set up the conditions that will enable us to introduce those changes into our organizations, rather than to have them imposed on us by outside forces. We must be willing to confront change openly, with breadth of vision. As managers we will have to play the role of a generalist rather than a technical expert; we will have to be the integrators, the synthesizers, the catalysts, rather than the ones involved with the nitty-gritty details of the job. Many managers have trouble making this transition—not only attitudinally, but in reality they are faced with increasing technological complexity in their jobs. The problem of delegating the more technical work to others while concentrating on the managerial aspects of their jobs is indeed a difficult transition for young managers.

A second major implication is that the manager of today had better develop an effective personal mechanism for handling stress. It is unlikely that anyone can remain in the mainstream of contemporary American business life and avoid a certain amount of stress and strain; in fact, studies clearly show that change and stress are related in a very definite way: The more change there is per unit of time, the more stressful it is for people. We can tolerate only so much novelty or unexpected change; we need routine and the expected.

Managers need to develop a way of handling stress that will enable them not merely to endure but to thrive in the world of change in which they will be working. It should also be mentioned that part of a manager's job is to help subordinates function well in the face of an increasing amount of stress in their lives. So managers have somewhat of a dual role: Although they must first look out for themselves, they must be concerned about the health of their employees as well, to prevent the widespread incidence in their workforce of some of the medical problems identified earlier.

REFERENCES

1. Judy Randle, "Coping with Stress," *Tulsa World,* April 23, 1978.
2. Hans Selye, *The Stress of Life* (New York: McGraw-Hill Book Company, 1976).
3. "Conquering the Quiet Killer," *Time,* January 13, 1975.
4. Kenneth Lamott, *Escape From Stress* (New York: Berkley Medallion Books, 1975).
5. Jean L. Marx, "Stress: Role in Hypertension Debated," *Science,* December 2, 1977, p. 905.
6. Ogden Tanner, et. al., *Stress* (Alexandria, Virginia: Time-Life Books, 1976).
7. Walter McQuade and Ann Aikman, *Stress* (New York: Bantam Books, 1975).
8. Kenneth R. Pelletier, *Mind as Healer, Mind as Slayer* (New York: Delta, 1977).
9. Alvin Toffler, *Future Shock* (New York: Bantam, 1970).
10. John W. Gardner, *Self-Renewal* (New York: Perennial Library, 1971).

CHAPTER 2

Understanding What Stress Is

Stress is a condition with which every human being is familiar, yet the term is so widely misused that it is often subject to confusion and ambiguity. Most people automatically assume that stress is bad; as a matter of fact, it may or may not be harmful, depending on the circumstances.

It is often useful to distinguish between what causes stress and what it is. The various pressures or demands from the external environment—which could stem from your family, job, friends, or the government—are called external stressors. The various pressures or demands from your internal environment are called internal stressors. They include the pressures you put on yourself by being ambitious, materialistic, competitive, and aggressive. In most of us, these internal stressors have far more intense an effect than do the external stressors. However, the important point here is that these external and internal pressures or demands are identified by the term *stressors*.

The bodily response to these stressors is what we call stress. Stress can be defined operationally in many ways. This book will use Hans Selye's definition: "Stress is the nonspecific response of the body to any demand."[1] It is now common knowledge that the human body has a stereotyped biochemical response to demands, whether pleasant or unpleasant. The stressors may be different, but they all elicit the same biological response.

The initial response to stress is very much like the basic alarm reaction of a person who is faced with the unexpected or with sudden danger. This response is often referred to as the "fight-or-flight" syndrome. Suppose you come home late one night after an extremely exhausting day at work. You are so tired that you have been hardly able to stay awake during the drive home. As you open your front door, you suddenly see flashlights inside and you hear hushed voices. Immediately and spontaneously, you become wide awake. A complex biochemical process has been set off in your body, and the following kinds of reactions occur: Photochemical changes take place in your retinas so that your eyes adjust to the darkness more quickly than they would have under normal circumstances; your hearing becomes momentarily more acute; your breathing and heart rates alter; blood rushes from the extremities to your chest cavity so that your vital organs will have all the blood necessary to operate at peak capacity; your brain wave activity goes up as extra supplies of blood rush to your head to allow your brain to function maximally; your muscles ready themselves for action.

What is happening is that your whole system has mobilized for action. If you decide to run, you will run more efficiently as a result of your system's being highly aroused. (You may remember what it was like to run scared when you were a child—you ran very well.) If you decide to stay and fight, you will fight better because of your body's state of preparedness. (You may remember fighting well as a child when you were really frightened.) However, the point is that upon sensing novelty in the environment—whether danger as in this case or some other form of the unexpected—your body automatically modifies itself to deal with the new situation. Your whole system becomes alive and alert, ready to respond as you see fit. Just as a country, when invaded, mobilizes itself to retreat or to advance and conquer, so the body prepares for action.

Here are some other examples of the fight-or-flight syndrome. Your boss calls you at home and says that he wants to see you, first thing in the morning, about something that is extremely critical to your future with the company. It doesn't matter whether you believe his news is going to be favorable or unfavorable; you may spend a restless night anticipating your conference. You will certainly have an initial stress response while talking on the phone, and you will have a similar reaction as you go into his office the next morning. The expectation of the event can be every bit as powerful a stressor as the actual event itself!

Or you have probably had the experience of nearly crashing into someone on the highway. If you are driving along and someone spins out in front of you and you have to swerve to avoid hitting the other car, you experience this alarm or emergency response.

Uncertainty and novelty are stressors. Anything which happens for the first time, or which you can't immediately make sense of, is likely to trigger stress. Normally, you quickly figure out what is going on or decide that it's not dangerous. Then the brain flips the "off switch" and the stress reaction stops before it becomes full-blown. If you can't figure out what's going on, but can find some constructive ways of handling the situation, the stress reaction will stop. But a full-blown stress reaction will be forthcoming if the danger is real and serious or if uncertainty and doubt continue on a prolonged basis.

Stress may be good for you

This fight-or-flight response may appear to be a good defensive reaction of the body. And that's true—the body's stress response is not only normal but essential! A fatigued body encountering danger will momentarily override its own exhaustion in order to deal with the danger. Obviously, this short-term stress is functional.

An important distinction to be made is that between short- and long-term stress. A composite of physiological data about yourself—including such factors as your resting pulse rate, muscle tension, brain wave activity, respiration rate, and level of sugar in the blood—will increase rapidly when you are experiencing short-term stress: Your body becomes sensitized and alert, ready to respond to the stressor. When you have coped with the crisis, this composite will drop dramatically, sometimes even below the theoretical baseline levels. Technically, this drop is called a parasympathetic rebound.

Claude Bernard, a French biologist of the past century, contended that the internal environment of our bodies must maintain a degree of consistency.[2] For example, blood pressure, heart rates, and oxygen levels are constantly shifting as a result of the demands of life. Yet the body cannot take too severe a change in these biological functions or allow them to persist too long without being damaged—or perhaps even dying. The work of Bernard was extended by Harvard physiologist Walter Cannon, who discovered that the body in its own wisdom triggers general adjustments when any change threatens to go too far. For example, when a person donates blood, multiple systemic changes in the person's body help compensate for the loss of blood: There are changes in heart rate and in blood vessels throughout the body, and fluid is transferred from tissues to the bloodstream. The body has numerous mechanisms to assist it in returning to a normal steady state, which is sometimes called homeostasis.

The "killer" form of stress is not short-term but long-term stress. Long-term stress consists of increasingly higher levels of prolonged and uninterrupted stress in which your system stays "hyped" up and never fully returns to baseline levels of activity. Gradually, over a period of time, your baseline may stabilize at higher and higher levels so that whereas a year ago your normal heart rate may have been 70 beats per minute, now it may have risen to 75–80 beats per minute. Blood pressure may increase in a similar manner, as may other biological functions.

Most managers deal with complex problems that defy simple solutions. The result is that we may fret over them for days on end. This may cause more stressors to develop, and the cumulative effect may be prolonged, uninterrupted, and increasingly higher levels of stress. According to Kenneth Pelletier, it is this prolonged, unrelieved stress that is primarily responsible for the development of the various stress-induced disorders.[3]

Elastic limits

The human body and stress can be compared to a spring. Imagine that we humans are springs of different sizes and shapes with differing tolerance levels, or elastic limits. Some of us can stand more stress than others, because we are made of "tougher material" or have been strengthened over the years to certain kinds of stressors. As long as we experience stress within our own elastic limits, we probably won't have any ill effects from it. But if we are pressed beyond our elastic limits, we may get "bent out of shape" and perhaps need to talk with a good friend or spouse to help us put things back together. If we are pressed far beyond our stress threshold to the breaking point, we may experience a complete breakdown, requiring professional help to restore ourselves to some semblance of normality.

Figure 1 illustrates how three different persons might have three very different threshold points and three different elastic limits. Person C can tolerate a greater amount of stress than Persons A and B before encountering the *yield point,* which manifests itself as a slight

Figure 1. Elastic limits.

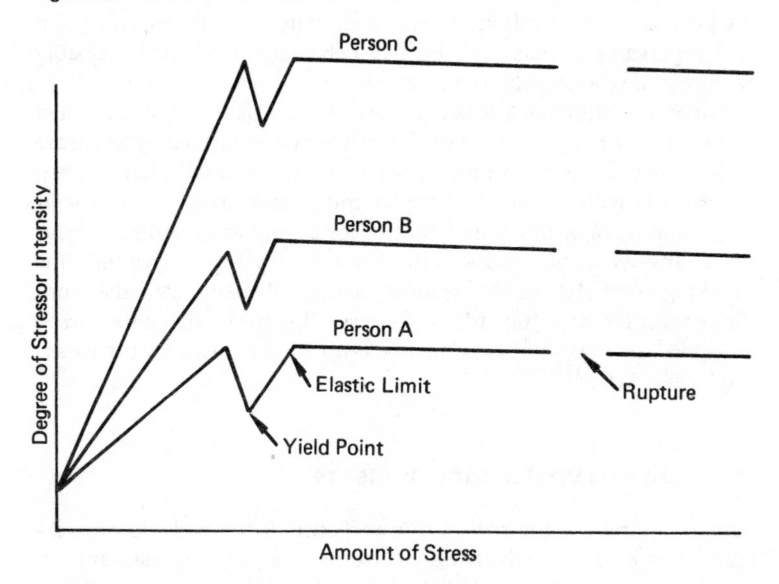

Yield Point = mild change from "normal" behavior
Elastic Limit = severe change in "normal" behavior
Rupture = Serious maladjustive behavior (nervous breakdown)

Adapted from Richard A. Morano, "How to Manage Change to Reduce Stress," *Management Review* (November 1977), p. 23.

change from "normal" behavior. The next critical point is called the *elastic limit*. In engineering terms, this is the point at which a stretched steel spring would begin to show deformation and beyond which the spring would not return naturally to its original shape. So it is with people: As long as the stressors are not intense enough to push us to our elastic limit, we thrive on stress. The yield point is a kind of early warning device that we are close to our limit, which could also be called our stress threshold. Only a slight increase in stress is needed to take us from the yield point to the elastic limit. For our purposes, we will say that as long as we are functioning within our elastic limits, the stress load won't be too great. However, beyond this stress threshold, we experience an increase in tunnel vision and rigidity. Figure 1 also indicates that if the stress load continues or intensifies once we are beyond the elastic limit, we will eventually reach the *rupture* point and experience serious maladjustive behavior, which will probably require professional help to correct.

In proper amounts stress is not necessarily bad for you. It is just like running a temperature. We all run a temperature as long as we are alive; it is only temperatures above or below "normal" that concern us. So it is with stress. As long as your stress load is within your elastic limits, or within your capacity for coping well, you will thrive on it. It's when you cross your threshold level and approach the breaking point that stress becomes distressful. Selye uses the word distress for the harmful variety of stress. "Eustress" (from the Greek eu—good, as in euphoria) is the made-up word he uses for the pleasant form of stress.

Pleasant and unpleasant stressors

Although stress is the nonspecific response of the body to any demand, it is irrelevant whether a stressor is pleasant or unpleasant; all that matters is the intensity of the demand of the stressor. An intense demand requires more of the adaptive capacity of the body and is thus more stressful than a mild demand. For example, the experience of being fired is very different from that of being promoted, yet in another way the experiences are quite similar. Receiving the news of being fired would be very stressful, because this message would in most cases be an extremely unpleasant stressor. Receiving the news of being promoted to a much higher position would also be stressful, because this message would be an extremely pleasant stressor. The specific results of these stressors would be very different, yet their stressor effect could be the same because of the stereotyped response of the body to *any* demand made of it. Of course, most people would find the firing more stressful simply because its negative effects might be longer lasting than the pleasant effects of the promotion. It could also be, as Selye emphasizes, that "eustress causes much less damage" because "it is how you take it that determines, ultimately, whether one can adapt successfully to change."[1] However, either the firing or the promotion could become distressful if a proper adjustment is not made rather quickly.

Differing degrees of stimulation can also produce different amounts of stress. "Deprivation or understimulation" and "excess or overstimulation" are both accompanied by increasing amounts of stress. Torture and brainwashing techniques have long capitalized on this understanding: To shut someone up in a small room for a long period of time with virtually no stimulation of any kind will drive the strongest of people insane. Likewise, to subject someone to a sensory barrage of flashing lights and loud noises of all kinds will also cause a person to snap.

We can also have too much of a good thing. Some people try to cram so much pleasure into their short vacation periods that they literally make themselves sick. People who are managing stress will monitor their pleasant stressors so as not to push themselves beyond their elastic limits, even if it means pacing themselves in having a good time. The would-be "playboy or playgirl" manager who works hard during the day at the office and equally hard night after night seeking social stimulation and excitement is risking trouble from distress. The body can't go at such a frenzied pace for long periods without suffering some damage. The damage may not always appear quickly, but the wear-and-tear impact of such levels of stress will be noticed and felt later on.

Stress threshold and recovery time

Differences in stress threshold levels and recovery rates are illustrated in Figure 2. Person B's stress threshold is just about twice that of

Figure 2. Stress thresholds and recovery rates.

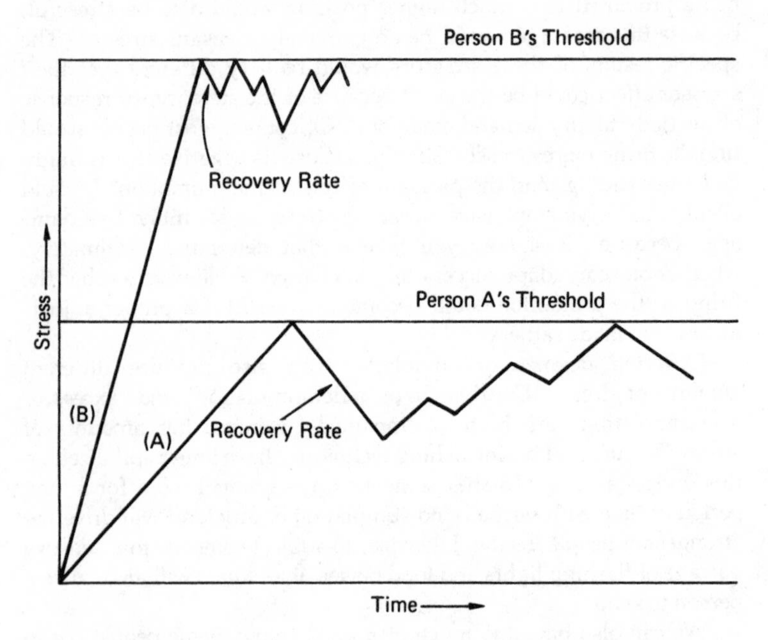

Adapted from Richard A. Morano, "How to Manage Change to Reduce Stress," *Management Review* (November 1977), p. 25.

Person A's. In addition, B's recovery rate is much more rapid. Person A feels the impact of a great amount of stress for longer periods, as indicated by the gradual slope of the recovery rate line as opposed to the steeper slope of B's recovery rate line. Thus, B can tolerate more stress within a given time period and can recover faster than A. Why some people bounce back faster than others can't be explained definitively, but it probably depends on heredity and past experiences.

Figure 2 also illustrates the cumulative effect of stress if it is allowed to build up over time without interruption. You'll recall that this long-term stress has the potential to be especially distressful if it is unrelieved. Sometimes rather mild-mannered people accumulate enough of a stress load from various sources over time that one additional, minor stressor may push them over their threshold level and cause them to explode unexpectedly. They get "bent out of shape," not by the triggering stressor or incident, but by the cumulative impact of multiple stressors pushing these people beyond their elastic limits.

Different stressors for different folks

What's very stressful for you may not be for others. For example, let's assume that you are in good enough shape to jog five miles a day, yet you never play tennis although you know how to play. You have a friend who is an excellent tennis player but who isn't in good enough condition to run five miles. Each of you is "in shape" for your own favorite sport. If your friend tried to jog with you for the full five miles, he might pull a muscle or even precipitate a serious medical problem, such as heat exhaustion or a heart attack; he would certainly be very sore the next day. Not being conditioned for such activity, he would definitely hurt his body in some way if he forced himself to run the entire distance, ignoring his body's signals to stop or to slow down.

On the other hand, if you got on the tennis court with him and really tried to match his performance, you would probably suffer physically because the abrupt, quick movements of tennis are very different from the movements associated with running. Being in shape for tennis is one thing; being in shape for long-distance jogging is quite another. This physiological example clearly illustrates the point: What is stressful for you may not be for others, and vice versa.

Specific experience with a stressor—be it physical or psychological—usually allows one to tolerate it better. With time, managers may become relatively immune to certain stressors. As has been pointed out, it's not the *intensity* of the stressor that determines how much of a reaction you will have; it's how you *react* to the particular stressor. Stunt men don't get hurt when they make long falls because they know how to roll with the fall. You and I would hit with full force—and we would get hurt, precisely because of the way we reacted.

So when problems arise, a manager who knows his company's system backward and forward, inside and out, may not respond in such a panicky way as the manager who is new to the company. The differences in responses of people to the same stressor may also be explained by genetic predisposition and by early family patterns of handling stress. Whatever the reasons, people do respond differently to common stressors. Of course, this fact makes the managerial job even more complex, because you can't assume that your people will be equally stressed by your managerial actions or inactions. How many times have you been taken completely by surprise by the reaction of one of your employees to some action of yours which you viewed as inconsequential? It is how other people perceive your behavior that will determine their reactions—not how you perceive it.

Some people appear to be cut out for the kinds of stressors generally found in managerial jobs; others are not. I know several persons who decided they wanted to go as far as they could in their career paths, yet stopped short of promotion into management. My first reaction to these people was to ask: "What's wrong with them? Why would they not be interested in being promoted into management with all of its additional responsibilities, challenges, and rewards?" On further reflection, however, I have often come to have more respect for this decision—some people would be better off *not* dealing with the particular stressors of managerial life. It is also true that some of these people might be shortchanging themselves because, given time and opportunity, they might eventually be able to adjust to managerial pressures.

Those who know their limitations and don't go beyond them are effectively countering the Peter Principle, which says that people get promoted to their own level of *in*competence and stay there. Time and time again, when an effective worker is promoted into management, his effectiveness as a worker is lost, and he often becomes an ineffective manager who is very stressed—a double loss. As a worker, the person was happy and productive; as a manager, he is unhappy, distressed, and unproductive. Yet the new manager feels that he can't go against the expectations of the whole society—his family, his boss, his company, and maybe even himself—and return to his lower-level job as a worker.

The process of selecting people for promotions is exceedingly difficult, and even when lots of time, energy, and care are put into it, mistakes will still be made. The answer in part to the Peter Principle is to correct selection errors once they are detected. This will take courage no matter who initiates it—the manager or the person involved. Yet, if one is truly not cut out for the managerial role, it is not unkind or harsh to urge that person to switch, or—if you are the person involved—to take the initiative and change jobs yourself. Once it is evident that the manager's job is not right for you or for one of your subordinates, taking such an action may prevent the stress from escalating to a point where it becomes distressful.

Stress and performance

The relationship between stress and performance is especially provocative for managers who are always interested in increasing productivity. The key to productivity is obviously in the performance of people. As Figure 3 illustrates, your performance and that of your subordi-

Figure 3. Stress and performance.

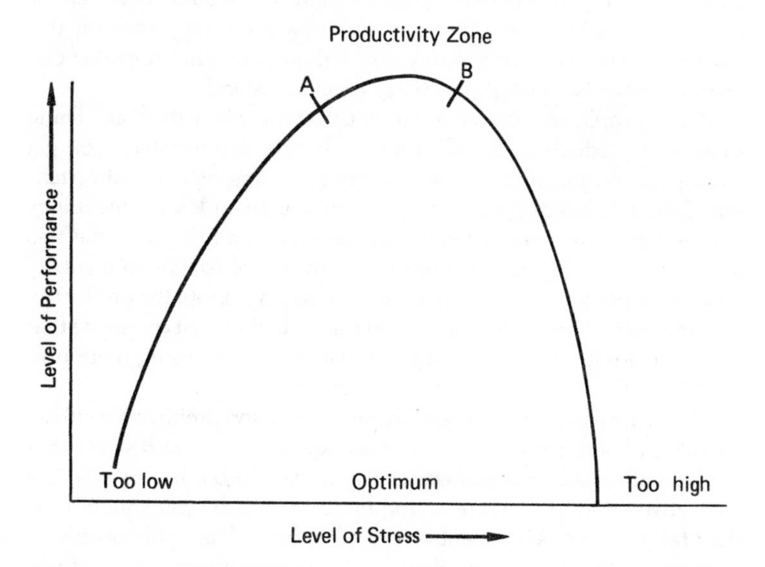

Adapted from Richard A. Morano, "How to Manage Change to Reduce Stress," *Management Review* (November 1977), p. 23.

nates is best when moderate demands (levels of stress) are being made upon you and them—if the demands are too low or too high, performance will be less than optimal. A simple example from sports will illustrate this point. At a critical point in the game, a basketball player steals the ball from his opponent and races down the court. The opposing team is in hot pursuit. The crowd is on its feet and is screaming at the top of its lungs. It is an extremely tense and exciting moment. Just as the player is about to go in for the lay-up, he kicks the ball out of bounds. What happened? The player was so keyed up and aroused (stressed) that his system was going faster than he could coordinate it, and therefore he lost control. According to Figure 3, he was on the downward slope of the inverted-U curve.

To illustrate the impact of too little stress on performance, think of the athlete who doesn't get himself "psyched up" for an important game. His lackadaisical attitude results in a rather lackluster performance. The superstars maintain nearly optimal conditions—a moderate amount of arousal (stress) in their bodies. A productivity zone is indicated on Figure 3 between points A and B. It would be unrealistic to expect an athlete or a manager to surpass the very apex on this inverted-U curve day in and day out, although it is not unrealistic to expect them to be in the productivity zone consistently.

Most people feel better about themselves when they are being somewhat productive. A dull, routine, boring day in which you get absolutely nothing accomplished is very discouraging and disheartening. Contrast that day with one in which you get at least some things done—there is a great difference in the way you feel about the two days. Occasionally, you may need to motivate yourself or your subordinates, or put yourselves under more stress, to get into the productivity zone. But whatever technique you use to do this, just recognize that you are not only doing your organization a favor by being more productive, but you will also feel better about it.

If you are a typical manager, the more common problem for subordinates and perhaps for yourself, is to experience so much stress that productivity is adversely affected. If you have subordinates who are ineffective because they are trying to do too much, you should consider taking some assignments away from them: They will not only be more productive employees; they will be happier as well. Also, if you are spreading yourself too thin, you might consider reducing your own workload through more effective delegation or through increased staffing. But for your subordinates or for yourself, it is important to be in the productivity zone. Of course, one of the chief indicators of whether people are beyond this zone and on the downward slope of the curve is their actual performance as measured by the criteria you normally apply to the work.

Motivation and stress

Motivation and stress are related. Motivating action often arises in an attempt to improve less then optimal conditions.[4] As the departure from optimal conditions becomes greater, your actions will usually become more powerful; as the departure from the optimum diminishes, your actions usually will become less powerful. Thus, stress would occur when your actions fail to reduce those less-than-optimal conditions. For example, let's say you are promised new offices for your newly hired staff as of September 1, but later you are told the offices will not be ready until October 1 and that you and your staff must manage to work together in one temporary office which is totally unsuitable. Conditions would be ripe for some action on your part. To the extent that you were successful in improving your office situation, your stress would lessen. If this were important to you and you failed to get the office ready on time or find better temporary offices, then you would most likely suffer from some stress.

Signs or symbols of departures from optimal conditions may stimulate action, and this helps explain anticipatory action. Similarly, stress may increase as one anticipates the stressful situation, and may actually diminish when that situation occurs. Reduction of stress may come as you discover that you have underestimated your ability to cope with the actual stressor. For example, you may dread an upcoming speech that you have to make. But the worst part may be the anticipation; once you're delivering the speech, your stress load will be much reduced.

Stress will increase not only when your threshold level is reached and you can't handle any more, but also when you are asked to tolerate some unpleasantness beyond what you are willing to endure. Using the example of the new office again, you might be able to tolerate doing without it for awhile, but you may simply be unwilling to do so. It is also true with this model that stress is likely to increase gradually rather than all at once. If the bad news about your offices were just one more in a long list of grievances, your stress reaction would probably be far more intense than if this incident were an isolated one.

Understanding motivation and stress is further complicated by the realization that you usually have several motives operating simultaneously. You may be coping very successfully with your immediate short-range goals, but suffering a great deal of stress because your long-range goals seem unattainable.

In defining motivation as an attempt to improve less-than-optimal conditions, A. T. Welford identifies three principles as the basis for a more precise meaning of "optimum."[4] First, people try to avoid extremes of stimulation, preferring to seek moderate levels. Both high levels of noise and complete lack of stimulation (sensory deprivation) appear to be distressing to human beings. Second, people prefer their stimulation to have moderate levels of predictability in both space and time: Both dull routines and continual unpredictable changes are disliked. Third, people prefer a moderate degree of conflict. Moderate conflict enlivens people; severe conflict is unnerving.

All three principles indicate man's need to find an optimum level of stress (arousal or stimulation). Welford has summarized it well:

> Sensory stimulation, novelty and conflict all tend to raise arousal level, while monotonous uniformity, predictability, and concordance tend to lower it. It is also well recognized that performance tends to be best at intermediate levels of arousal: the organism is insensitive and inert if the level is too low, and tense and disorganized if it is too high.[4]

By thinking of "optimum" in this way, you can see that human capacity applies to more than muscular strength. Performance is less likely to be hindered by physical limitations than by the time necessary to resolve uncertainty in making decisions, the amount of data that can be handled at once, or by time pressures. When people are below optimum levels of performance, they are underactive, and their mistakes are mainly errors of omission. When people are above their optimum level of performance, they are overactive, and they make errors of commission. As Welford has put it, "Monotony and boredom resulting from too little demand tend to produce an inert type of performance and a tendency to drowsiness, while the tension and anxiety that accompany too great a demand often lead to rash and ill-considered actions, lacking due caution and restraint."[4] It is also true that the optimum level is lower for more difficult tasks than for easier ones.

REFERENCES

1. Hans Selye, *The Stress of Life* (New York: McGraw-Hill Book Company, 1976).
2. *Stress* (Chicago: Blue Cross Association, 1974).
3. Kenneth R. Pelletier, *Mind as Healer, Mind as Slayer* (New York: Delta, 1977).
4. A. T. Welford (ed.), *Man Under Stress* (New York: John Wiley & Sons Inc., 1974).

CHAPTER 3

The Manager Under Stress

The sources of stress in today's world are many and varied, although whether it is more stressful to be living now than in earlier times is open to question. In all likelihood, psychiatrist Karl Menninger is correct when he says, "the difficulties of adjustment to the stress and strain of contemporary living have been bemoaned and deplored for every generation since long before the Christian era."[1] It is more important to confront and examine what the stressors are in our lives. This is a necessary first step in finding ways of reducing stress to manageable levels. When you recognize a stressor and know what is affecting you, you are in a far better position to choose wisely among the various stress-reduction techniques to help you deal effectively with your stress. Because similar stressors often make different individuals respond quite differently (based on individual circumstances, heredity, and physical and emotional makeup), it is very important that you be honest in your attempts to analyze what is "bugging" you and what the stressors are in your own life.

It is often assumed that managers and executives are more vulnerable than nonmanagers to the ravages of stress. Although the harassed, ulcer-ridden, overly tense executive does exist, he isn't as common as is generally believed. In fact, some have pointed out that executives tend to get healthier as they move up the corporate ladder, and most middle managers with lots of responsibility and never quite enough authority to cover that responsibility have more problems with stress than do executives. These top executives may have a relatively low rate of heart attacks and suicide precisely because they have survived the ordeal of climbing the corporate ladder.

When he was chairman of the Medical Board of the Life Extension Institute, Dr. Harry Johnson studied some 25,000 executives and came to the conclusion that executives as a whole are a healthy group.[2] What this means is that although ulcers are commonly thought to attack busy managers more frequently than the average citizen, the evidence does not support this conclusion, and there appears to be no special health hazard that comes from being a businessman or manager. A sprinkling of ulcers is found at all levels of responsibility in organizational life. No one is immune, and greater responsibility does not appear to lead to health problems. As Dr. Johnson has put it: "It's not what a man does between 9 A.M. and 5 P.M. that poses a health hazard—it's what he does from 5 P.M. to 9 A.M. that we're concerned about." Dr. Johnson obviously is convinced that the totality of your life must be considered when you are examining the impact of stress upon yourself.

A study done by Laurence E. Hinkle, Jr., and his colleagues at Cornell University Medical College has exploded the myth that rapid advancement in industry and high levels of responsibility are associated with an increased risk of heart attack. Hinkle's study was based on a five-year survey among 270,000 men in the Bell System throughout the United States. Every incident of coronary heart disease that occurred among these men was examined. The researchers concluded that the rates of coronary heart disease are higher among men who are *not* in management, and that the rates actually declined at each step up to a higher level of the organization.

You must be careful not to jump to any conclusions as a result of the above data. It would certainly be a mistake to assume that the more promotions you get the more likely you personally are not to suffer from coronary artery disease. We must remember that statistics deal with collective numbers. They are not predictive of what may happen in any one individual case. What the above information really means is that you simply can't single out the manager, and particularly higher levels of managers, and say that they risk being a special health hazard because they are managers.

Sources of stress

The conceptual model in Figure 4 presents a classification of sources of stress at work and how these stressors interact with characteristics of individual and extraorganizational sources of stress. These interacting variables lead to symptoms of excessive stress and ultimately to disease. Studies in experimental laboratory settings[3] and in the workplace[4] are part of a growing body of evidence strongly suggesting that occupational stress is indeed a causal factor contributing to the kinds of disease discussed in Chapter 1. Using this model, we will identify various stressors that managers commonly face.

Environmental stressors at work

The model divides the possible environmental sources of stress at work into five categories: factors intrinsic to the job, role in organization, career development, relationships at work, and factors associated with the organizational structure and climate.

FACTORS INTRINSIC TO A JOB

Each job has sources of stress which are integrally connected to that particular job's requirements. In addition, all jobs have certain common stressors. In this section we shall explore six of these stressors: boredom, poor physical working conditions, time pressures and deadlines, exorbitant work demands, information overload, and job design and technical problems.

Boredom. You probably remember having a job about which you said, "I am bored to death." Although it is very unlikely that anyone has ever died of actual boredom, it is quite true that boredom can be an important factor in inducing sickness. A major study[5] made by the University of Michigan's Institute for Occupational Safety and Health, and by the U.S. Department of Health, Education, and Welfare (HEW) found that boredom may produce stress as fast as, or perhaps even faster than, the traditional killers of the Industrial Revolution—long hours, heavy workloads, and pressing responsibilities. In this study, the researchers questioned men in 23 occupations ranging from factory work to university administrator. A questionnaire

Figure 4. Sources of stress at work and their consequences for the individual.

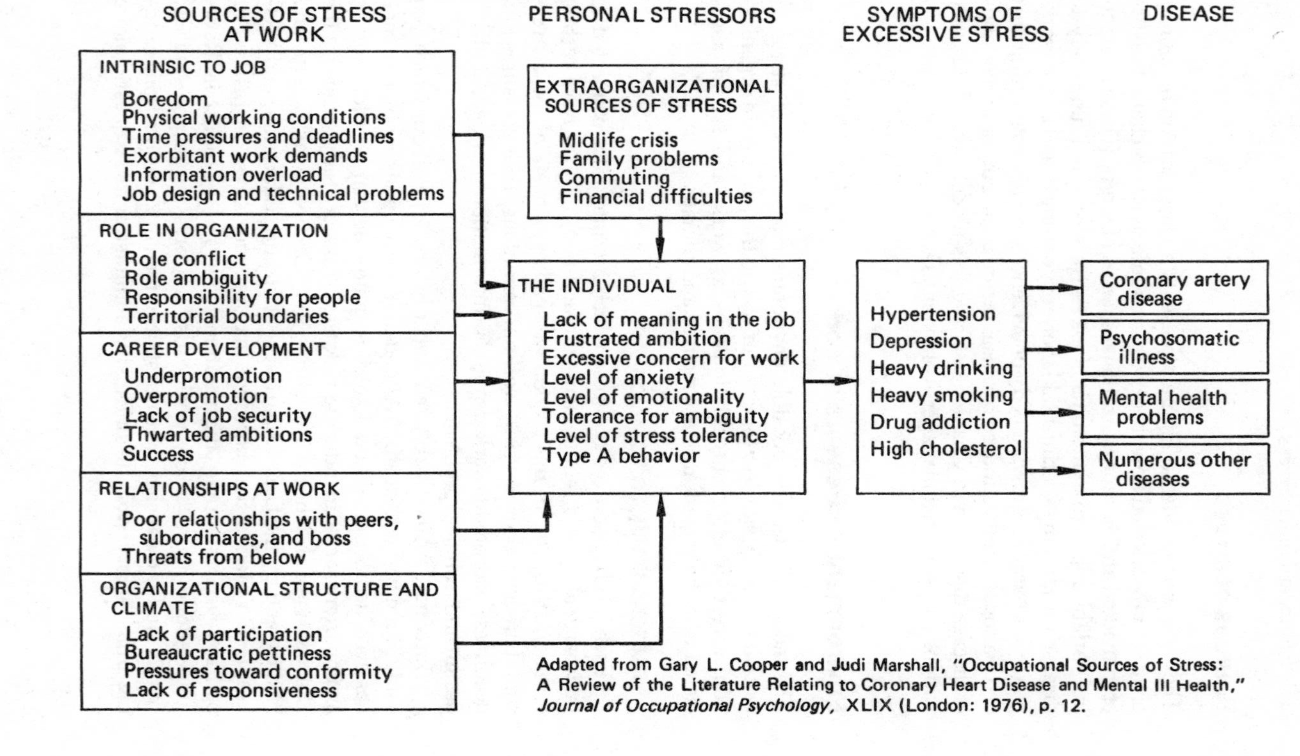

Adapted from Gary L. Cooper and Judi Marshall, "Occupational Sources of Stress: A Review of the Literature Relating to Coronary Heart Disease and Mental Ill Health," *Journal of Occupational Psychology*, XLIX (London: 1976), p. 12.

was administered to 2,010 men employed in these jobs, and physiological data such as blood pressure, heart rate, serum cholesterol, thyroid hormone, serum uric acid, and serum cortisol were collected from 390 men in 8 of the 23 jobs.

Workers who reported both the most boredom and the greatest dissatisfaction with their workload were the assemblers and relief people on the machine-paced assembly line. Symptoms of stress—such as anxiety, depression, and irritation—were also highest among the machine tenders and the assemblers and relief people on the assembly line. The study concluded that employees who report a high degree of boredom in their work are likely to feel that their skills and abilities are not being used well, to rate their work low in complexity, and to have a poor fit between the amount of complexity they want and the amount that their jobs provide.

According to Dr. Harry Johnson, fatigue is often emotional in origin, and is related to boredom.[2] If you are suffering from extreme boredom, you are very likely to start work in the morning feeling bad and not having any energy for your work. You are not interested in your work, because it presents no challenge. More rest isn't the answer for this form of fatigue; somehow you must renew your interest in your job or find other interests or outlets—or perhaps another job.

Recently I was talking with a colleague about the new legislation concerning mandatory retirement. He said, "I don't think this new legislation attacks the right problem. The real problem in this country is that people get bored with what they are doing. No one can avoid boredom or becoming "burned out" on a job they've been doing for 20 years. We need a different law—one which says that nobody can work at the same job for more than 20 years." In other words, he was suggesting that there be a mandatory shifting of jobs every 20 years in order to prevent a person from becoming bored and dissatisfied and probably unproductive on the job. I suspect that he was rather clearly indicating how he felt about his own work. Nevertheless, as surprising as it may seem, boredom is a major stressor for many people in this country, managers and workers alike. Even among professionals, you hear them worrying about "professional burn-out." Call it what you will, boredom is a serious drain on productivity in this country.

Poor Physical Working Conditions. Two of the conditions that are most often associated with poor physical working conditions are noise and crowding. Jerome E. Singer and David C. Glass have summarized four important principles that seem to be at work in how environmental stressors such as noise and crowding affect us.[6]

First, most environmental stressors are not intense enough to cause *immediate* physical damage. The discomfort is felt immediately; however, the physical impact of the stressors is cumulative and long range.

Second, the social and emotional context of an environmental stressor is as important as the physical properties of the stressor itself. When you are on your own turf, crowded and noisy conditions don't have the same impact upon you as when you are on someone else's turf. A noisy, crowded family reunion in your home is quite different from a noisy, crowded affair in a stranger's home.

Third, people are amazingly adaptable. Whether it be to extremely crowded conditions or to high noise levels, in time most of us are able to adjust satisfactorily.

Fourth, particular psychological or social factors can ease or aggravate the effects of an environmental stressor. For example, it has been found that people can work under rather adverse conditions and, unless pushed too far, can hold up well under such conditions as loud noise or even crowded office conditions. However, many times those employees who work under noisy, crowded conditions are less efficient and are less tolerant of frustrations *after* work than those who can do their work in more favorable conditions.

How environmental noise can bother people in this indirect after-effect fashion has been studied extensively, and three general environmental characteristics that serve to soften these after-effects have been identified:[6]

1. If the noise or crowded condition occurs with predictable regularity or if it can be anticipated, it will not be as harmful as if it is unpredictable. You are far more likely to get upset as a result of a traffic jam at 2:00 in the afternoon on a major freeway than if it were to occur at 5:30 P.M. The reason, of course, is that you expect heavy traffic conditions at 5:30 but not at 2:00. Studies clearly show that unpredictable noise almost always produces more detrimental after-effects than predictable noise; in fact, soft unpredictable noise is worse than loud, predictable noise.

2. The social context in which environmental stressors occur is of great importance. If you are trying to prepare your new budget be-

cause you are facing a pressing deadline, the sound of a nearby typewriter can be rather annoying. However, your annoyance may be far greater if the person operating the typewriter is someone else's secretary rather than your own.

3. By far the most important factor is a feeling of control (or the lack of it). In a fascinating study, Singer and Glass compared the ability of two groups of workers to tolerate irritating levels of noise.[6] One group worked under noisy conditions but was given the option of pressing a button if the noise became too irritating; the other group did not have this option. Most of the people in the first group completed their work without pushing the button. When their work output was compared with that of the second group, it was found that those who worked in the noisy environment without the button made errors on reading tasks and arithmetic problems, showed little tolerance of frustration, and were unwilling to do favors for other people. People in the other group who worked under equally adverse conditions, but who *did* have the option of pressing the button, showed almost none of these after-effects. The reason for the difference in productivity is quite clear: People in the latter group believed they could press the button and stop the noise if they chose to do so, and as long as they believed they had this option (even though the button would not actually work), the results would be the same. As has been mentioned earlier in this book, your perception of reality is the basis for your behavior even though reality may be somewhat different from your perception of it.

The importance of the feeling of being in control was also confirmed by researchers in Stockholm, Sweden, who studied the stressful effect of going to work by train.[1] The researchers found that even though passengers who got on the train at the beginning of the line traveled for an hour and 40 minutes, they experienced considerably less stress than passengers who got on midway and traveled for only 50 minutes. The researchers used the "feeling in control" concept to explain this curious phenomenon: Passengers who boarded the train early had far more control over where they sat, with whom they sat, and how and where they arranged their personal belongings than those who boarded the train when it was almost full. Thus, you may be able to tolerate greater amounts of physical stress if you also feel that you are more in control.

Time Pressures and Deadlines. Almost by its very nature, your managerial job throws you in the midst of time pressures and deadlines. You only have to be reminded of how stressful deadlines can be. The urgency of deadlines is real; it is even bound up in the word itself, which evokes an image of a line beyond which lies—death! During periods just before deadlines, the pressure builds up rapidly. But once the deadline is met, everyone feels greatly relieved.

It is not uncommon for a manager to experience the pressure of deadlines in such a way as to question whether he is in control of his life or whether his watch and calendar are controlling him. I once heard a chief executive say that the one piece of equipment he owned that he couldn't do without was his watch. If you have ever had to do without your watch for several days or have lost your calendar indicating all of your appointments for the next week, you know just how stress-provoking this can be. Whenever I ask managers to identify key stressors in their organizational life, time pressures and deadlines are always at the top of the list. So it is rather evident that time pressures constitute one of the key stressors intrinsic to a job.

Exorbitant Work Demands. Exorbitant work demands—tightly scheduled work days, heavy travel, and simultaneous demands—can also exert considerable stress. These demands can crowd your days so that you are not able to get your paperwork done in the office. As a result, you may take the paperwork home and create additional stress there.

The reasons for exorbitant work demands vary, although one of the most common is understaffing. One executive vice-president was so overworked that when his job was finally fully staffed, it took three additional people to do the work that he had been doing all by himself for several years. During that time he had been working late at night and every weekend, probably putting in 70- to 80-hour weeks!

Another reason for exorbitant work demands is simply that your business may be a cyclical one characterized by peaks and valleys: When the peaks come, you work very hard for a short period of time; but then the valleys appear and you can slack off. The peak periods may not be distressful to you, even though they are stressful—especially if you know that there are valleys ahead.

Information Overload. In any one day, most of us are exposed to far more information than we can adequately digest and absorb. As a result of the availability of the copying machine, friends send us copies of articles and reports and ask us for our reaction to them. We would just as soon file them in the round file, yet because of friendship, we often feel compelled to glance at the reports so that we can have some reaction for our friends. In addition to this information, most managers feel the responsibility to read the daily newspapers, certain management journals, technical journals in their primary discipline, relevant memos that cross their desks, and general correspondence. At no time is it more evident to us just how much information does come across our desk on a daily basis than when we go on vacation for two weeks and return to the office to face the stack of paper that has accumulated in our "in" basket. Just as overstimulation at the sensory level increases the likelihood of our distorting reality, so cognitive overstimulation, or information overload, may interfere with our ability to think and to process information in order to make sound decisions.

Job Design and Technical Problems. Some jobs are by nature very stressful. Air traffic controllers at large airports have a heavier stress load than most people, because their decisions have to be right and the stakes are very high. Dealing with irate customers is usually stressful until you have done it for a while: How would you like to tell airline customers who have their tickets in hand that their flight was overbooked and that you don't have a seat for them, even though they have tickets? How would you like to be the customer relations representative at the local Social Security office who must calm down the irate citizen who didn't receive his or her check that month? These jobs, like many others, are inherently stressful. Yet as we get used to them, the stress may be greatly reduced.

Other jobs are potentially stressful because the work is interdependent with someone else's work. For example, you may not be able to get your work done on time because you're waiting for some critical part which the procurement department failed to order in time. As a result you may miss the deadline on an important project, and although it won't be your fault, your boss may still hold you responsible for that failure.

In engineering and in other technical fields, jobs are often stressful because of the technical problems they present. (Stress may be created by uncertainty about which decision is technically superior.) A manager in a technical field is often expected to keep up with "state of the art" technology in his field—*and* to be an effective manager. This double role can be a real burden.

ROLE IN ORGANIZATION

Another primary source of stress at work is your particular role in the organization. Conflict and ambiguity about your role can take its toll in increased anxiety and decreased productivity. The amount of responsibility you have for people and the territorial boundaries inherent in your managerial role can also be key stressors.

Role Conflict. Role conflict as a source of stress in organizational life probably has been studied more extensively than any other single organizational stressor. In general, the studies over the years have tended to indicate that people who suffer more role conflict have lower job satisfaction and higher job-related tension than those who don't experience so much role conflict. According to Daniel Katz and Robert L. Kahn, role conflict is "the simultaneous occurrence of two (or more) sets of pressure such that compliance with one would make more difficult the compliance with the other."[7] Katz and Kahn describe four kinds of role conflict: (1) intrasender conflict, (2) intersender conflict, (3) interrole conflict, and (4) person–role conflict.

An example of *intrasender* role conflict is when your boss asks you to complete a particular project by a certain deadline, yet at the same time he or she makes the impossible demand that you go through all the proper channels, not missing a single signature you must obtain. In this particular example, your boss has asked you to achieve two objectives that are in apparent conflict: If you do go through all the proper channels, you know that you will not complete the project by the end of the day; if you complete the project, you know that you cannot go through all the proper channels: Thus, you feel as if you are in a bind—the essence of role conflict, be it intrasender role conflict or any other form.

Intersender role conflict is prevalent with matrix organizations. The essential organizing principle in a matrix organization is that you report to a department manager functionally but at the same time are assigned to one or more special project leaders. In this case, a conflict may very easily arise between your department manager who gives you your performance reviews and your project leader to whom you are temporarily assigned for a special purpose. You may very well find yourself in a bind on a particular day, not knowing whether to please your department manager or your project leader, both of whom have legitimate authority over you.

Interrole conflict occurs when two different roles that you assume in life are in conflict. For example, when you are fulfilling your role as a businessman by traveling, you can't be home to fufill your role as family man. At that moment the two roles are at loggerheads.

Person-role conflict occurs when your organization expects you to assume a particular role or roles that are in conflict with your own basic values. For example, a certain aerospace engineer, whom I shall call "Joe," is approximately 45 years old, was educated at one of the military academies, is a very good engineer, and has been one all his working life. In the last 10 to 15 years, he has entered engineering management, and is widely recognized as a very competent technical person as well as a good manager. He is at the stage in life where his family is making peak financial demands on him: Two of his three children are in college, and he has an expensive home in a surburban area. And yet this man has a very serious problem—he has recently "gotten religion." For Joe, "getting religion" means that all of a sudden he has become a pacifist. He no longer believes in military work, even for defensive purposes. Thus, he finds himself in a serious conflict. His value system is in conflict with his work role, and the only thing he has ever done in life is to design and build weapon systems. Joe is paying the price for this conflict in a very physical way—a year ago, he almost died of a bleeding ulcer. Joe's situation may be a little dramatic, but is probably not as atypical as you might think. Indeed, role conflict in any of its various forms is certainly a source of stress in organizational life.

Role Ambiguity. Role ambiguity is another major organizational stressor. It is usually thought to exist when you have an inadequate amount of information about your role at work and where there is a lack of clarity about the objectives of your position, about colleagues' expectations of your work role, and about the scope of responsibilities of the job itself. The effects of role ambiguity upon people generally parallel those of role conflict. Most studies indicate that people who suffer from role ambiguity experience lower job satisfaction, higher job-related tension, a greater sense of futility and perhaps even lower self-confidence than those who don't have such an ambiguous position.[8] Individuals seem to differ vastly in just how stressful they find role ambiguity to be. By virtue of their experiences, some people may even thrive on the ambiguity; others demand a high degree of structure in their lives and find ambiguity very upsetting. The organization also must play a role in just how stressful an individual may find role ambiguity. When the stakes are high, role ambiguity is most pernicious. When people in organizations are most protective and supportive of their employees, ambiguity appears to be more tolerable, and perhaps even preferable. As people in jobs are given more autonomy and freedom it should not be surprising to find more ambiguity in their job descriptions.

Responsibility for People. In a major study done at NASA's Goddard Space Flight Center, John R. P. French, Jr., and Robert D. Caplan, found that the more responsibility a manager had for people (as opposed to things), the more likely he was to encounter stress.[9] French and Caplan defined responsibility for people as including their work, their careers and professional development, and their job security. Responsibility for things was said to include budgets, projects, and equipment and other property. The administrators, engineers, and scientists at Goddard who had greater responsibility for people than for things spent large amounts of time interacting with people in meetings and on the phone, and had much less time for working alone. They also reported that they spent a great deal of time under deadline pressure, often to the extent that they could barely keep up with their routine work. The people in the study who had more responsibility for things than for people had little or none of these adverse effects. Thus, in an organization, a significant source of stress may be responsibility for people. Managers who have greater responsibility for people than for things are more likely to experience stress than their counterparts.

Territorial Boundaries. It is generally felt that territorial boundaries are as important to people in organizational life as they are to animals in the wild. Human beings seem to develop feelings of ownership regarding their own offices or their own particular line of work, and will fight aggressively to keep others from violating their own "turf." If we all do feel more comfortable in our own territory, this raises the question of what the stress impact is on an individual who has to interface extensively with departments other than his or her own, and what is the impact on people of having to work in a department alien to their home base. The Goddard study cited above has explored these two variables, and the researchers have found that individuals who interface extensively with departments distant from their own usually had lower self-actualization values and lower utilization of their best abilities and leadership skills, whereas those who spent most of their time with people in their own work units had a higher level of self-actualization.

As might be expected, it was also found that people who worked in an alien environment showed more stress than those who didn't. For example, administrators who worked in an engineering unit showed more symptoms of both quantitative and qualitative overload, greater deadline pressures, higher systolic and diastolic blood pressure, and a faster pulse rate. Likewise, engineers who were working in an administrative unit displayed greater deadline pressures, more contacts across organizational boundaries, less opportunity to do the kind of work they preferred, less opportunity for advancement, and lower levels of self-actualization. Organizational boundaries are real and they define territory; and although they are often desired by the people involved, protecting such boundaries can have an adverse stress effect. Thus, organizational boundaries can be another important source of stress in organizational life.

CAREER DEVELOPMENT

A third set of environmental stressors at work is related to career development, or how well you are progressing in your chosen career path. Advancement is an extremely important matter for many managers. Problems in career development (underpromotion, overpromotion, job insecurity, thwarted ambition) and sometimes even success itself can contribute to high stress levels.

Underpromotion. If you have ever been on a job in which your abilities were not being well utilized, I am sure that you will not need to be convinced that underutilization of abilities or underpromotion is a major source of stress in careers. A rather poignant story is told by Gerald J. Soltas about his experience with underutilization:

> When I was released from the service, I was looking forward to finally getting a chance to be a "real engineer." I guess you could say I was gung ho. I took a job with a large shipyard in Virginia that had several contracts to build navy warships. I had almost four years of sea duty as a missile fire-control and systems officer, and I felt I could apply my education and experience to building those ships and their missile systems. It

was a rude shock to me when I was assigned to antisubmarine systems about which I knew very little.

It was worse to realize a few weeks later that I wasn't expected to know or do very much. I read more than one novel and many magazines just to have something to fill the hours. I was not alone in my frustration, either. Numerous other engineers referred to their time-filling activities as "making eight." To compound the aggravation, we were occasionally required to put in overtime because "the project was behind." Talk about waste! A master's degree in automatic control systems engineering, four years of experience on the navy's newest missile systems, and I was reduced to checking plans from some jerk in Washington who probably had never seen the inside of a college or ship.

It really got to me. I was coming home from work frustrated and discouraged. I've never been particularly easy to get along with, but my wife said I was becoming even more of a grouch. I had to do something![10]

As Andrew J. DuBrin points out, creating stress for people by not using them well is rarely the result of a conscious plot by the higher-ups in organizations; it often happens simply because it's difficult to find a good match between human resources and job requirements, and because there are often not enough challenging and exciting jobs to go around.

Overpromotion. Overpromotion is a term that is sometimes used to describe a person who has reached the peak of his abilities and has little possibility for further career development and yet may be given responsibilities that exceed his capability. This phenomenon has been called the Peter Principle, in which a person will rise to his appropriate level of *in*competence and will tend to stay at that level. If you are at your level of incompetence and yet are being asked to do work beyond your capacity, it is almost certain that you will be suffering from excessive stress. You may or may not be aware of it, but there is a strong possibility that you are suffering a great deal of inner turmoil as you struggle to keep your head above water. You may expend a lot of energy denying that you are in this position, or covering it up, or perhaps even driving yourself hard in order to be able to handle your increased responsibilities.

Selecting people for jobs is one of the most difficult managerial tasks any one of us will ever have. We usually have to select people for a new job based on how well they have performed on a previous job, which may be totally different from the new one that we have in mind. We would see less evidence of the Peter Principle in organizations if more managers had the courage to correct selection mistakes once they realize these mistakes have been made. This failure to act on our part is more of a problem than the phenomenon of the Peter Principle itself. Yet being overpromoted undoubtedly puts you in a rather stressful position, particularly if you are not able to grow fast enough to handle the new tasks. Whether you stay with the new task or let yourself be moved down to a lower level, there is a great deal of stress involved.

Lack of Job Security. In the aerospace industry, it is common knowledge that a sense of job insecurity does not drive you to work more productively, but rather puts you under so much stress that you become ineffective in your work. Under these conditions, people might be expected to work harder at their jobs in order to be among the last to be laid off; however, studies indicate that people actually spend a great deal of their time on coffee breaks and at the water cooler discussing who will be laid off next. Abraham Maslow and many other psychologists have made us aware of the importance of a sense of job security as a minimal condition for productive work. I use the word "sense" because it is your *feeling* that's the important thing. You may actually have very little security at work; but if you *feel* you do, then your behavior will be more influenced by this feeling than by the actual circumstances.

Thwarted Ambition. If you are now several managerial levels below where you had expected to be by this time in your career, you are likely to experience a fair amount of stress as a result of your disappointment. No matter what their cause, thwarted ambitions—particularly for highly ambitious people—are quite stressful. We need to sense progress in the development of our careers. One study done among U.S. Navy personnel resulted in three interesting conclusions: (1) Navy personnel experienced greater job satisfaction when their rates of advancement somewhat exceeded their expectations; (2) dissatisfaction increased as advancement rates slowed down; and (3) those who were least successful in advancing tended to perceive the greatest amount of stress in their lives.[8]

Success. As strange as it may seem, success can be very stressful for some people. When you are successful once, others will expect you to be successful again in the future. You may also expect it of yourself or feel the need to match the expectations of others. This pressure to be successful can be so great that you or your subordinates may actually avoid success! Here, though, you should remember that stress in proper amounts can be good for you. The reason some people are successful is that they keep the pressure on themselves at least to match their past performance. As long as this stressor—or pressure, isn't excessive, it can be extremely functional in helping you advance in your managerial career.

The above set of environmental stressors related to career development are only suggestive and are representative of the kinds of stressors that you or others may face. Our careers are intensely personal, and success in our careers has a great deal to do with the way we feel about ourselves. Thus, it should not be surprising that frustrations in career development are likely to be stressful for all of us.

RELATIONSHIPS AT WORK

The relationships you have at work are potentially a source of eustress or distress. You have probably known people who were extremely excited and "high" about their work (eustress) because of the quality of people with whom they were working; undoubtedly, you also have known people who were literally made ill because of their associations at work. In a celebrated case, Baxter Ward, one of five supervisors for the County of Los Angeles, was accused by Philip Watson, the county tax assessor, of having "caused" his heart attack by constant harrassment. Whether such was the case would be hard to prove, yet Watson surely believed it to be true.

Difficult relationships at work can bring on symptoms associated with extensive stress such as diarrhea, pain in the neck or lower back, anxiety, and insomnia. Certain associates can *literally* be a "pain in the neck." A man whom I shall call Harry used to have a completely disruptive effect on the entire headquarters staff every time he came in from the field. Harry was very bright, aggressive, and idealistic. He had absolutely no patience with incompetence or even with human error. Harry could not understand why the system didn't operate perfectly. Every time he came in from the field, he left frustrated, anxious, trembling lower-level employees and upset, irritable higher-level employees in his wake. When Harry had been to headquarters, you knew it—you could see the human damage. Harry was a major stressor for a large number of people—his subordinates, peers, and superiors.

When you choose a new job or when you are considering hiring someone new, a big consideration is how good you expect your relationship to be with the people involved. You don't want to move to a new job where your arrival will create strains among the people there, nor do you want to hire someone who will disrupt your already existing good relationships. Many behavioral scientists believed that good relationships at work are a key factor in both individual and organizational health. Most of us are probably able to confirm this belief from our own experiences.

In the Goddard study at NASA, French and Caplan identified the quality of relations that people have with their supervisor, peers, and subordinates as a key organizational stressor.[9] They defined poor relations as those that involve low trust, low supportiveness, and low interest in listening to and dealing with problems. They discovered that poor relations were often the result of role ambiguity, inadequate communication, and role conflict. Once established, poor relations tend to produce psychological stress in the form of low job satisfaction and belief in the existence of job-related threats to a person's well-being. Poor relations with subordinates do not seem to affect feelings of being threatened whereas poor relations with peers and with your immediate supervisor do affect the threatening feelings. Thus, threatening feelings are more likely to be reduced by improving relations with peers and with your supervisor than with your subordinates. Autocratic, demanding bosses do put you under stress. This stress may be justified in the short run, yet it's still stress, and you may not like it even though you have to put up with it.

Another source of stress found in relationships at work is the threat that may be posed to you by the arrival of, say, some rising star just out of Harvard Business School who has just been put into your department. You begin to get anxious. "He'll have my job before long," you may think. "I'll bet he knows much more about management than I do. I'm sure top management is grooming him to take my job and move me to the side." All these feelings are understandable, although probably inaccurate. You're probably overestimating his ability and selling yourself short. You're not giving yourself any credit for the valuable insights you've gained from your experience with people over the years. You also know far more about your company's politics and its established methods of getting results. In short, you may have no real need to worry, but you worry anyway. You begin to feel inferior. Others, including your boss and the specific person from below who represents the threat, start to notice the feelings of inferiority that you manifest in your behavior. Before you know it, the inevitable happens—he or she does get your job! And *you* are primarily responsible for the result. It was a self-fulfilling prophecy: By feeling inferior, you *acted* inferior, and pretty soon you really *were* inferior.

At times, there will certainly be legitimate threats from below, yet you probably shouldn't interpret all threats as legitimate. To the extent that you sense this threat, it will be stressful to you. Of course, this stressor could stir you to needed improvements, or it could be the beginning of the end—but that is primarily up to you.

ORGANIZATIONAL STRUCTURE AND CLIMATE

The organizational structure and climate is another important source of stress at work. In any organization you must give up some of your freedom and individuality in order to be a part of the system. But in addition to this fundamental fact of organizational life, there are other related stressors: lack of participation, bureaucratic pettiness, pressures toward conformity, and lack of responsiveness of the organization.

Lack of Participation. Not having the opportunity to participate in decisions that affect your job is another organizational stressor. We all like to influence decision-making processes that affect our way of doing our work. Of course, many times we couldn't care less about participating in decision making, because it may not affect us, or perhaps we don't care how a decision goes. Yet we feel differently when we do care about the decisions.

French and Caplan have summarized the findings of a number of separate studies on the effect of low participation on employees: "Of all the stresses we have considered, low participation has the greatest harmful effect on job satisfaction and threat." Thus, it appears that your sense of psychological well-being may be strongly influenced by the amount and quality of your participation in those decisions closely tied to important aspects of your work.

Figure 5 summarizes the findings of French and Caplan regarding characteristics of persons who participate in decisions that affect their work.

Bureaucratic Pettiness. Every organization of any size has a myriad of rules, policies, and procedures that make sense only to the person who created them. There may have been problems that arose because of a lack of a specific procedure, so several procedures and rules were created to cover a situation that probably would occur only with the greatest infrequency. Ridiculous rules, policies, and procedures constitute one form of bureaucratic pettiness which you may face.

Another common form of bureaucratic pettiness is represented by the classic line, "That's not in my job description," or "Another department takes care of that." When you are trying to get something done, these two responses can be quite stressful, and are indicative of the pettiness which characterize bureaucracies that have become "bureaupathological," i.e., sick organizations.

Pressures Toward Conformity. Pressures toward conformity are real—though often subtle—in organizational life. Some organizations are noted for demanding conformity of dress and behavior, but the most dangerous and shortsighted conformity is in the area of ideas. Pressure to buy U.S. Savings Bonds may result in 100 percent participation by the employees, and this result should be satisfactory to those concerned. Yet some executives also want their employees to actually *think* that U. S. Savings Bonds are one of the best financial investments they could possibly make.

Although this example of thought control may be relatively harmless, it can be stressful for some, and is certainly not very farsighted on management's part. Irving Janis has documented the potential danger of what he calls groupthink—the "striving" for agreement so characteristic of highly cohesive groups.[11] Groups which don't permit divergent thinking are the weaker for it, because they become so insulated that they may lose touch with pertinent realities in their environment.

In recent American history there is no better example of the intense and powerful demand for conformity in an organization than the White House Staff during the Nixon administration. Using "national security" as a rallying cry, members of the President's inner circle—

Figure 5. Characteristics of persons who participate in decisions which affect their work.

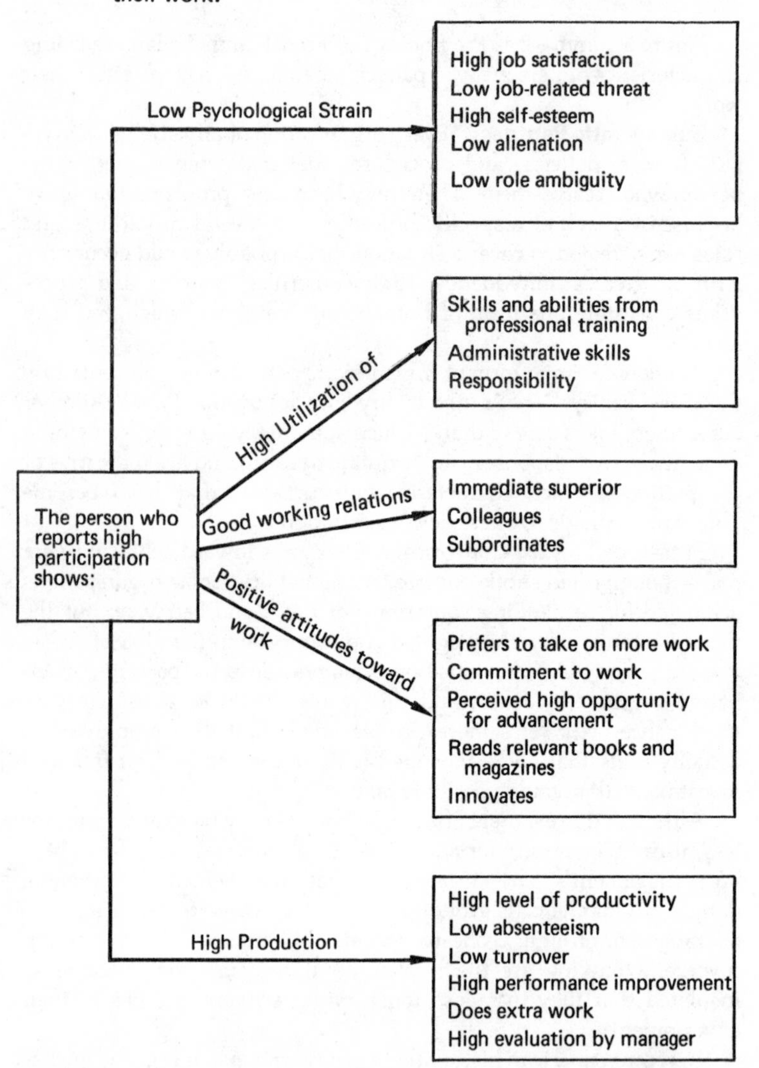

Adapted from: John R. P. French, Jr. and Robert D. Caplan, "Organizational Stress and Individual Strain," *The Failure of Success.* Ed. Alfred J. Marrow. (New York: AMACOM, 1972), p. 52.

H. R. Haldeman, John Ehrlichman, John Mitchell, Jeb Magruder, and John Dean—committed criminal acts out of a twisted sense of loyalty to the administration. The Watergate investigations revealed the tremendous pressure that these men were under (and that they exerted on each other) to be "team players" and do whatever the President told them to do—no matter how reprehensible the deed.

Lack of Responsiveness. A particularly damaging organizational stressor is when the upper echelons of management are simply unresponsive to the requests and reports of lower-level employees. Nothing seems to bother people more than just being ignored. We appear to prefer any response—even a negative one—to no response at all. Not only are people distressed when they are met with unresponsiveness; they are also discouraged from taking any initiative in the future. Why should they make the effort if they don't even get the courtesy of a response?

While doing management seminars for a major "think tank," I asked the scientists to name the number one stressor in their work. They unanimously picked the unresponsiveness of management. I have repeated this question many times in workshops and, without exception, management's lack of responsiveness is always identified as a major stressor—it doesn't seem to make any difference what kind of work the organization is doing or whether it's in the public, private, or not-for-profit sector.

Personal stressors

In the model we are using to define stress, the organization is only one of three major ingredients; the other two consist of personal stressors —stressors that pertain to your personality, and those that arise from sources other than your work or your personality, but are intensely personal nevertheless. For convenience, we shall divide personal stressors into these two categories: the individual and extraorganizational sources of stress. Conceptually, the model suggests that organizational and extraorganizational stressors are conditioned by your own personality: You may respond very differently than someone else would to the very same organizational and extraorganizational stressors. For example, you may work well under deadline pressure, whereas someone else may make mistakes and get very upset. Problems that arise from rearing a teenager may bring you many headaches, whereas someone else may find it easy. The difference is primarily in your response. No one else in the world could respond as you would, because you as an individual are unique. But before we discuss how your personality determines your reactions to various stressors, let's first explore some extraorganizational sources of stress.

EXTRAORGANIZATIONAL SOURCES OF STRESS

This category comprises personal stressors that do not arise exclusively from your work or from your individual personality but that are related to both. Although extraorganizational sources of stress are generally experienced as personal problems, they are problems that are not unique to you and are not directly of your own making. These stressors include the midlife crisis, family problems, commuting difficulties, and financial problems.

Midlife Crisis. In recent years, a great deal has been written about what has been variously called the male menopause or the midlife crisis. Lee Stockford of the California Institute of Technology has indicated that five out of six men in professional or managerial positions undergo a period of crisis in the middle years as they compare who they are with who they had hoped to be by this time in their careers. He says that one out of every five men who undergo this crisis never fully recovers from the shock.[12] People who do not recover go through the rest of their lives bitter and cynical, complaining about politics or about a particular person who blocked their career advancement.

The midlife crisis typically occurs somewhere between the ages of 35 and 45, although it can occur earlier or later. Let's take "Jim," a typical manager, 40 years old, who is going through a fairly typical midlife crisis. Jim progressed well in his career up to this point. He now has enough data about himself to assess how far he is likely to go up the corporate ladder. He has probably not reached his peak, but he can see the extent of his success. Jim starts to ask himself questions: "What's it all about? What are my real values? What is important to me? Why am I pushing myself to get ahead?" Like many others facing the midlife crisis, Jim may very well decide that his family is the most important thing to him—the family that he has neglected for the past 10 to 15 years as he worked so aggressively to get ahead in the corporate world. Sadly enough, Jim's renewed interest in his family is probably too late: His family is now relating more and more to the outside world. Jim's wife, who has been at home with the children for the past 16 years, has suddenly developed a new interest in a career of her own—just as Jim's interest is turning inward toward the family. She no longer has time to take the weekend family trips and outings that she had been urging Jim to go on for years. Jim's two boys, who are now grown teenagers, are no longer interested in engaging in various activities with Dad; they would rather be with their friends. Needless to say, Jim is a little chagrined and troubled because the members of his family have grown away from him—just when he feels a desperate need to engage them more deeply than ever before.

Over the past few years, a very personal sense of mortality has been developing in Jim. It started five years ago when his grandparents died, and has intensified recently with the unexpected death of his 65-year-old father. Jim has also known some colleagues and friends who have died unexpectedly at the age of 40. This personal preoccupation with death was exacerbated by Jim's realization that his own life was more than halfway over. His growing sense of his own limits and mortality is causing Jim to reexamine his values.

In reëxamining his values, Jim's attention is likely to focus first of all upon his wife. He has been married to her for 18 years. Recognizing that his life is more than halfway over, he tries to assess whether she is the person with whom he wants to spend the rest of his life. After 10 to 15 years of marriage, many couples start to take each other for granted. In Jim's case, this has also been true, and he begins to explore whether he is still in love with his wife. There may be a few turbulent years ahead for him and his wife as they examine their marriage more deeply than ever before, trying to decide whether they can bring mutual satisfaction to each other now and throughout the rest of their lives. Divorce is by no means inevitable, although there are many divorces during the midlife crisis. But if Jim's marriage survives these turbulent years, it has a very good chance of becoming even stronger than it has ever been.

Jim may also think about the particular company for which he is working, and he may assess his own particular job. This, of course, is done in the context of clarifying his values in all areas of life. Jim may decide that he does not like his long commute (40 miles, one way) and that he wants to spend more time with his family, more time in recreational activities such as tennis, and more time with friends. It would not be at all surprising to see Jim change jobs, if not careers, in order to maximize time for the things that he has now decided are of utmost importance to him. Abrupt career changes as well as job changes are often made in the midlife crisis.

Another manifestation of this crisis may be Jim's wish to cut his ties with his mentor. As Jim progressed up the corporate ladder, he had a mentor who provided guidance and counsel, which at the time was most helpful. But in the last few years, Jim has decided that he has got to break that tie, lest he maintain his dependency upon the mentor. This cutting of the tie can be traumatic, because Jim feels a tremendous sense of loyalty, obligation, and appreciation for the one who has counseled him in his career and who has helped him through critical phases of it. Nevertheless, he now feels the need to be his own man.

Sexually, Jim may begin to experience some frustrations as the aging process begins to take its toll upon him. He may find it difficult to meet the renewed sexual interests and desires of his wife who, in her late thirties, is now sexually at her prime. As problems develop in this particular area, Jim's reaction to them will determine how much more stressful they will become.

All in all, the midlife crisis can be as turbulent as the identity crisis of adolescence, but as with any crisis there is always an opportunity for growth and development. If Jim handles this crisis well, he will derive greater fulfillment and growth from it.

Family Problems. Your family has the potential of being either a source of relief from stress or a source of stress itself. It's probably not surprising to recognize that when stress occurs excessively at home, it can be very upsetting. Traditionally, home is supposed to be a place where you can truly be yourself and find understanding, acceptance, support, and love. Whether a home approaches this ideal depends largely on the quality of the relationships among the family members. In no way am I trying to suggest that normal or even ideal families don't have problems and that in these homes there aren't feelings of anger and resentment. There obviously will be negative feelings from time to time. However, there should also be a commitment to share these feelings regularly so that they can be aired and not allowed to build up over time into even deeper resentments. The positive commitment to understand and accept even negative feelings will ensure the continued love and support of everyone.

Nevertheless, it's still true that when tensions and worries about any family problem are high, there will inevitably be lots of stress. The most common family problems center on money, sex, child-rearing practices, and communication (usually a lack of it). Everyday living in a family setting brings with it plenty of stress. Minor misunderstandings, insensitivities, and problems are the "stuff" of which any normal family life is made. Family problems can affect your work adversely: It's just not possible to keep your family concerns (especially major ones) from affecting other areas of your life. What's important is to regularly monitor the stress gauge on you and your family and to control the stress level by dealing with it openly and directly.

Commuting. Perhaps no other stressor connected with urban life is so devastating as is commuting to and from work. If you've ever commuted very far, it won't be hard to convince you of this. Some researchers studied the connection between stress and heart disease in a number of top executives in various lines of work.[1] The researchers attached pulse counters to the subjects' wrists and asked each of them to note what activities they were involved in throughout the day, so that these activities could be plotted against the pulse rate. One of the subjects was a newspaper editor who commuted daily by automobile from the suburbs to San Francisco. All the researchers expected his peak pulse activity to come as a result of emergency crises at work, such as the presses breaking down at an inopportune moment. But they were startled to find that his most stressful activity throughout the day was commuting to and from work! Of course, it should be noted that the effect of this stressor, as with any other, is only partially determined by the intensity of the stressor itself; how you respond psychologically to it is just as important. If you learn not to get "uptight" about your commute, it won't be as stressful for you as for the person who just can't sit back and take it in stride.

Financial Difficulties. Living above one's means is almost as American as apple pie. In your efforts to acquire more and more material goods, you may be putting a great deal of extra pressure or stress upon yourself. You may end up working longer and harder hours trying to get that promotion, or you may work a second job or send your spouse to work. Even if you do nothing but worry, the course of action you take will affect other areas of your life and will add to your burden of stress. For example, putting your spouse to work undoubtedly will create some new strains in your marriage. Moonlighting and working harder, longer hours would take a heavy physical toll that could adversely affect your other roles simply because of a lack of physical stamina and energy. Financial difficulties are particularly stressful, because we usually take them very personally: Your ego may be so deeply involved that you will take it very hard, feeling that it reflects on your ability to earn the money that you and your family need. Thus, it's quite easy to see why financial problems rank as a major stressor in many lives.

Many other extraorganizational sources of stress could be identified, including social relationships and the tensions resulting from living with day-to-day international news as reported in the press and over radio and television. You are encouraged to reflect on your own personal situation and to identify your own personal stressors in this area.

THE INDIVIDUAL

You as an individual interact with all these different stressors, and your reaction to them will be determined in part by your feelings, values, and unique personality characteristics. Six of the most common of these "individual" stressors are discussed here.

Lack of Meaning in the Job. Ideals have a greater impact on us than we may acknowledge. We desire jobs that have meaning and relevance. Of course, you usually decide for yourself whether your product or service is socially relevant. DuBrin offers two very different perspectives by two toy designers. The first design engineer says of his job, "What a way to spend my working days. I'm simply adding fuel to a waste economy. How purposeless to design new and better toys for children. I think they would be better off playing with pots and pans."[10]

The second design engineer with the same job puts it quite differently: "I'm glad my job is a useful one. Think of all the young minds

I'm helping to develop as they play with these creative toys. Not only am I giving children an opportunity for enjoyment, but I'm helping them grow intellectually."

Obviously these two engineers are poles apart in their view of their jobs as toy designers. To try to determine who is right is to miss the point; how each one *feels* about his job is what really counts. You probably can find some significance in almost any job, although there is more in some jobs than in others. Yet when you find yourself feeling that your work has insufficient meaning, you are very likely to become stressed. You may even change jobs in an attempt to find one with greater meaning.

Frustrated Ambition. If by this time in your career, you had planned on being several levels higher in management than you are now, and if this goal had been and still is very important to you, you are likely to be frustrated. Most of us gradually accept the inevitable and adjust to it in time. Some of us must lower our expectations, while others must raise them. Of course, settling for less of a position than you'd desired often leads to frustration.

The essence of frustration is to be blocked by some barrier from reaching your goal. It's bad enough to fail to achieve our objectives when something or someone external to us is the reason; it's even harder to take when the reason for our failure is our own inadequacies. But whatever the cause, when you as an ambitious person are hindered from reaching a vitally important career or job goal, you are going to experience some degree of frustration. This frustration will become more and more stressful unless you accept reality or find a way to get around the barriers that keep you from your goal.

Obsessive Concern for Work. In your drive to get ahead, you may become obsessed with work. You may attempt to achieve your ambitions by putting in longer hours and working harder and harder. In many cases, you may find this technique self-defeating because you may become less effective due to the long hours you're working. You've so diluted your time, energy, and interests that you find it hard to focus on any activity for long because of all the competing demands.

You would probably be far better off working "smarter" rather than just harder. Peter Drucker makes an interesting distinction between efficiency and effectiveness. Effectiveness comes with doing the right job well, i.e., doing the tasks associated with your job that you alone should do because of the unique contribution you can make based on your particular strengths.[13] Efficiency results from smooth operations, but the tasks being smoothly operated in a businesslike way may or may not be the ones that are important for you to be doing. Obsessive concern for work may result in a decline in both efficiency and effectiveness, although it's more likely that effectiveness will be curtailed.

Many managers believe that the way to move up is to take on more and more work and to efficiently handle all that they can. Yet my observation is that managers more often get ahead by being effective in turning a visible critical activity from a losing one into a profitable one. Developing the ability to concentrate on the few key activities to be accomplished is the better way to move ahead in your organization.

Level of Anxiety. Some of us are more anxiety-prone than others. A common dictionary definition of anxiety calls it the "painful or apprehensive uneasiness of mind usually over an impending or anticipated ill." Anxiety often involves the feeling of not having ways of responding appropriately to the anticipated harm. Anxiety usually is experienced as a sense of edginess, apprehension, and dread.

Often, there are understandable reasons for feeling anxious. Personal factors such as illness and family problems may contribute to it, as may organizational factors such as frequent changes in administration (which can make you feel uncertain about your own position); the intense competition for a limited number of upper management slots; job ambiguity and pressure; lack of job feedback; and job insecurity because of volatility in the economic environment.[14]

As with stress, you should recognize that all anxiety is not detrimental to health. In fact, moderate anxiety can be functional in mobilizing and focusing your energy on finding innovative solutions to problems. It's when anxiety is severe and prolonged that it can cause you to be distressed and thus less functional.

The extent to which you get anxious will depend upon the intensity of the anxiety-producer and your own personal make-up. If you are subject to a free-floating anxiety that can be activated by the slightest suggestion of harm, then you are likely to suffer much anxiety. For you, a well-structured job with clear-cut tasks would be desirable.

Another person who is not particularly anxiety-prone could better tolerate a job without much structure.

Level of Emotionality. Emotionality refers to the emotional make-up that underlies individual differences in emotional stability; changeability in moods; tendencies toward guilt, worry, anxiety, and lower self-esteem; sensitivity to environmental sources of stress; concern about physical health; and experience of tension. Neuroticism is the more technical term for the emotionality dimension of a person, but because it may connote maladjustment, it will not be used here.

A certain level of emotional arousal is necessary for learning and performance. Too little or too much arousal, however, will adversely affect learning and performance. Some of us are "by nature" higher on the emotionality index than others. If you score high on such an index, you will "require less externally induced motivation to reach the level of emotional arousal optimal for performance." Under such circumstances, you could also "withstand less intense external motivational pressure" before your performance deteriorates. However, if you score low on the emotionality index, you may require a lot of external pressure before you get "in gear."[14]

These studies clearly indicate that if you are high in emotionality you will be especially susceptible to the stressful effects of role conflict and role ambiguity, and particularly when strong pressure accompanies the role ambiguity. In your managerial role you can minimize the stressful effects of role ambiguity and role conflict by providing supportive supervision for your subordinates who are high on emotionality—that means lots of positive feedback and a minimal amount of pressure from you. Individuals who are high on emotionality are not undesirables; they are as loyal as any, and you can get them to maximize their production and satisfaction by treating them appropriately. (Of course, subordinates who are low on emotionality will need more pressure from you.) Differences in individuals necessitate different approaches.

Perhaps you're wondering how to identify who among your subordinates is high on the index of emotionality, or just how *you* might rate on such an index. The simplest way is to observe behavior. Hamner and Organ summarize it this way: "Frequent references to guilt feelings about trivial matters, expressions of worry about health that seem exaggerated or unconfirmed by medical examination, a habit of working feverishly to complete minor projects long before their deadline, obsessive concern with possible traumatic events in the distant future, inability to shrug off past mistakes or failure, are all possible clues."[14]

Tolerance for Ambiguity. Stress caused by ambiguity about one's role in an organization was discussed earlier in this chapter, and at that time it was indicated that people differ in their tolerance of such ambiguity. Of course your own personality makeup will largely determine how you will respond to job ambiguity. Many researchers believe that a tolerance for ambiguity will increasingly become a vital characteristic of the manager who successfully moves up the corporate ladder. As the bulk of the labor force continues to shift from production jobs into what Peter Drucker calls "knowledge worker" jobs, there is the strong probability that a greater percentage of jobs will be characterized by somewhat fuzzy job descriptions. So the challenge of role ambiguity is liable to be even greater in the future than in the present. It will be interesting to see how this trend develops and whether these conditions will increase our ability to tolerate ambiguity.

Level of Stress Tolerance. Individuals vary tremendously in their capacity to deal with stress. Even what is perceived as stressful will be different to different individuals. This individual variation in level of stress tolerance is, of course, an important mitigating factor in the model proposed here.

Type A Behavior. The work of cardiologists Friedman and Rosenman was briefly mentioned in Chapter 1. Their research over the past 20 years has led them to the conclusion that the person with a Type A personality is two to three times more likely to suffer from coronary artery disease than is the Type B personality.

The essential characteristics of Type A people are that they have a chronic struggle with time, always trying to do the most they can do in the shortest amount of time; they are very competitive and aggressive; and they usually have some sort of undirected hostility lying just below the surface, waiting to be provoked. Type B people have some of these same qualities, but the qualities are not chronic, incessant, or constantly overdone.

It is believed that roughly half of the American population consists of Type A personalites, probably because of the puritan ethic and a socioeconomic system that has consistently rewarded many of the values associated with Type A behavior. All of us have some mixture of Type A and Type B in us, but one is usually dominant. Obviously, the purer the Type A behavior, the more dangerous it could be for you, but some words of caution are necessary here. First, being a pure Type A does put you in a statistically more dangerous group, yet you *as an individual* might never have a problem with heart disease; statistics only tell us of probabilities in groups and nothing definite for any one person.

Second, because we all vary in our ability to tolerate stress, some of us may be constitutionally better equipped than others to handle Type A behavior. The concept of *elastic limits,* presented in Chapter 2, is pertinent here. Some of us may be able to display Type A behavior without harm as long as we don't go beyond our elastic limits—even Selye states that some people are race horses and others are turtles. He means that some of us must move fast to be ourselves, whereas for others a much slower pace is necessary. Just as a race horse not allowed to run and stretch its limbs will deteriorate quickly, so a pure Type A person would probably suffer if he or she had to follow a Type B behavior pattern. However, in light of the medical findings, if you do have a pure Type A personality, you might consider pulling back a bit, just to be on the safe side, because you may not know precisely what your elastic limit is.

The work of Friedman and Rosenman was initially viewed with a good deal of skepticism by the medical profession, which did not like the idea of cardiologists dabbling in "psychology." However, today, after many years of thorough research, most medical doctors are convinced that Type A behavior is a major risk factor in coronary heart disease. Friedman and Rosenman's research has typically been longitudinal (10 years in one study) with adequate sample sizes (3,500 in one study) and sound research designs, often "stacking the deck" so as to make it improbable that Type A behavior would be singled out as a major factor.

By filling out the questionnaire on page 67, you can determine to what extent *you* have Type A behavior. Rate yourself on a scale of 0–10, with 10 being extremely high and 0 extremely low. Consider 5 to be an "average" person's response to each of the questions. Thus, for Question 2, if you consider yourself average on moving, walking, and eating rapidly, you would put a 5 in the blank by that question. When you finish answering the questions, add up your ratings. If you score higher than 60, you are likely to have a Type A personality. Common sense must be used, since this form can't precisely indicate your behavior pattern, and it assumes that you know yourself well and that you also know what constitutes the "average" person's basic behavior pattern—neither assumption may be correct. You might get a friend or a spouse to confirm your score. (I am indebted to Drs. Friedman and Rosenman for some of the concepts that I have incorporated in this questionnaire.)

Drs. Friedman and Rosenman's technique is to interview people and then rate them more on their actual behavior than on what they say. For example, the doctors will ask a simple question very slowly, so that when they're half-finished asking it, the question will be obvious. Type A people will usually interrupt and answer it before the questioner has finished.

Let me give you a few examples of Type A behavior that I have personally encountered. My own wife Carolyn from time to time displays such characteristics. For example, one day several years ago I came home from work and went upstairs into the children's bathroom where she was with my 11-year old daughter, Camille. As I walked in, I noticed that she was doing something to Camille's hair which I had never seen done before, and I heard her counting out loud very rapidly from one to twenty. I looked at her in a very puzzled way and said, "What in the world are you doing?" "This is a curling iron and I am curling Camille's hair," she responded. "The instructions say to hold this lever down and count slowly to ten, but I can't count slowly, so I am counting to twenty, fast." This is a perfect example of the tendency of Type A people to move rapidly in everything they do. Whenever I speak in public and Carolyn is in the audience, she loves the speech no matter what its content—as long as I speak rapidly; however, if I slow down too much, she finds it very difficult to follow and to applaud, no matter how good a speech it might have been.

One of the best examples of Type A behavior is that of my friend whom I shall call John. John is a very successful businessman who has his own insurance business. Because John's busy week begins on Monday morning, he drives frantically to work, aggressively jockey-

SYMPTOMS OF TYPE A BEHAVIOR

	Rating
1. To what extent do you hurry the ends of a sentence or explosively accentuate key words even when there is no real need to do so?	_____
2. To what extent do you always move, walk, and eat rapidly?	_____
3. To what extent do you feel impatient with the rate at which most events progress and openly exhibit your impatience to others?	_____
4. To what extent do you strive to think or do two or more things simultaneously?	_____
5. To what extent do you always find it difficult to listen to those who don't especially interest you?	_____
6. To what extent do you always feel vaguely guilty when you relax and do absolutely nothing for several hours to several days?	_____
7. To what extent do you no longer observe the more important or interesting or lovely objects in your environment?	_____
8. To what extent do you attempt to schedule more and more activities in less and less time?	_____
9. If you meet another severely afflicted Type A person, to what extent do you find yourself compelled to challenge him instead of feeling compassion for him?	_____
10. To what extent do you resort to certain characteristic gestures or nervous tics?	_____
11. To what extent do you believe that your success is due in good part to your ability to get things done faster than anyone else, and are you afraid to stop doing everything faster and faster?	_____
12. To what extent are you increasingly committed to evaluating in numerical terms not only your own behavior but also the behavior of others?	_____
Total Score	_____

ing for position on the freeway. He actually has timed the stop lights on the boulevard he uses to get to his office, so that when he exits the freeway he knows exactly how fast he has to go in order to make all the lights! I feel sorry for you if you get in his way. John pushes himself all week, working late hours and scheduling as many appointments in a day as he possibly can. He keeps himself keyed up throughout the week, rarely sleeping well at night because of it. Friday night he spends partying, and all day Saturday he plays as much tennis as he possibly can. He goes to another party Saturday night (and by the way, at parties John is totally capable of dominating the conversation). By Sunday afternoon, John's system is finally fatigued enough that it forces him to stop and collapse. He tells me that he gets one great night of sleep each week—Sunday night—and then he is up and at'em again Monday morning.

One of the purest Type A personalities I have ever met, John is a prime candidate for coronary artery disease, especially since his family has a history of the disease. John is successful in business as a classical Type A person, but you should not assume that Type A people are always more successful than Type B people. There are many successful Type B people (although they do have a lot of Type A's working for them—in order to get a lot of work done in a short amount of time!).

The cause of Type A behavior is not fully known, although traditionally it has been thought to be genetic. However, Friedman and Rosenman contend that Type A behavior patterns are just as likely to be learned at a very early age in the primary family relationship. In their opinion, this may explain why coronary artery disease tends to run in certain families: It may be the *family behavior patterns, not* the genes, that are transmitted from one generation to another.

Regardless of the cause of Type A behavior, it should be pointed out that people can and do change from Type A behavior patterns to the safer form of Type B. Friedman and Rosenman recommend a program of modifying your behavior through rewards and punishment. One example they give relates to the tendency of Type A people to run a red light in order to save time. If you desire to change this behavior pattern, they suggest that you make a pact with yourself so that the next time you run a red light you make yourself come back around the block. Obviously this is a form of extreme punishment for

Type A people, because they are always in a hurry. If you are faithful to your pact, you will discover pretty soon that you actually save time by stopping for the red light. This act of stopping becomes a reward in itself because instead of losing time and punishing yourself by having to take the block again, you will actually save time. Although it does take willpower to follow through on such a program, a carefully thought out program of behavior modification can be extremely effective in changing your own behavior pattern from that of Type A to Type B. In doing so, you will put yourself in a lower risk group for coronary artery disease.

The rest of the conceptual model illustrated in Figure 4 suggests that a person under heavy stress from organizational and extraorganizational stressors may eventually display certain common symptoms of excessive stress before he or she manifests any of several stress-related diseases. Your individual make-up will have much to do with whether any ill symptoms appear and, if they do, which particular disease you may contract. (Specific diseases that may arise because of distress were discussed in Chapter 1.)

REFERENCES

1. Ogden Tanner, et al., *Stress* (Alexandria, Virginia: Time-Life Books, 1976).
2. "Advice to Businessmen on Health and Retirement," *U. S. News and World Report,* March 7, 1966.
3. Robert L. Kahn and Robert P. Quinn, "Role Stress," *Mental Health and Work Organization* (Chicago: Rand McNally, 1970).
4. Bruce L. Margolis, William H. Kroes, and Robert P. Quinn, "Job Stress: An Unlisted Occupational Hazard," *Journal of Occupational Medicine,* October 1974.
5. Robert D. Kaplan, et al., *Job Demands and Worker Health: Main Effects and Occupational Differences* (Washington, D.C.: U.S. Department of Health, Education, and Welfare, 1975).
6. "Making Your World More Livable," *Stress* (Chicago: Blue Cross, 1974).
7. Daniel Katz and Robert L. Kahn, *The Social Psychology of Organizations* (New York: Wiley, 1966).
8. Gary L. Cooper and Judi Marshall, "Occupational Sources of Stress: A Review of the Literature Relating to Coronary Heart Disease and Mental Ill Health," *Journal of Occupational Psychology,* March 1976.

9. John R. P. French, Jr., and Robert D. Caplan, "Organizational Stress and Individual Strain," in Alfred J. Marrow, ed., *The Failure of Success* (New York: AMACOM, 1972).
10. Andrew J. DuBrin, *Human Relations: A Job Oriented Approach* (Reston, Virginia: Reston Publishing Company, Inc., 1978), pp. 71–72.
11. Irving Janis, *Victims of Groupthink* (Boston: Houghton Mifflin, 1973).
12. Harry Levinson, *Executive Stress* (New York: Harper & Row, 1966.)
13. Peter Drucker, *The Effective Manager* (New York: Harper & Row, 1966).
14. W. Clay Hamner and Dennis W. Organ, *Organizational Behavior: An Applied Psychological Approach* (Dallas: Business Publications, 1978), p. 202.

CHAPTER 4

Danger Signs and Symptoms of Stress

Many people are able to see how excessive stress is adversely affecting other people's lives, but fail to gauge its impact on their own situation. It's very much like the situation of the alcoholic, who is usually the last to realize that he or she is indeed an alcoholic. This failure in self-awareness is quite understandable in the context of American managerial culture: Managers who rise to executive levels are known for their aggressiveness, their drive, their initiative, and their ability to handle pressure. As President Truman once put it, "If you can't stand the heat, get out of the kitchen." Given this set of values, are you likely to admit very easily that you can't take being in the pressure cooker any longer? It's doubtful that you'll admit it to your boss or yourself, lest you end up facing a demotion or—at the very least—almost no chance for further advancement. So, before dismissing the possibility that you, too, may be under excessive stress, ask your spouse or a good friend whether he or she observes in you any of the danger signs described in this chapter.

You should remember that a certain amount of stress is necessary to energize your system, to tune you up and keep you alert and ready for what life may bring. Yet, when you go beyond your own natural limits, certain predictable negative bodily reactions will eventually occur. There are medical indications of stress which you and I can't observe, such as the blood levels of adrenalines, corticoids, ACTH, and certain white blood cells called eosinophils. Nor are you likely to have the necessary equipment to check your cholesterol level, your brain-wave activity, your blood pressure, or the electrical conductivity of your skin. However, there are plenty of signs that you *can* observe, some of them more serious than others. For convenience's sake, these danger signs will be divided into four categories: (1) the general adaptation syndrome; (2) danger signs at work; (3) rate of life changes; and (4) Selye's list of danger signs and symptoms. In some discussions of stress, the general adaptation syndrome is dealt with when defining stress itself; however, I have chosen to discuss it separately because the manifestations of the syndrome constitute some key warnings of stress.

The general adaptation syndrome

While stress is the nonspecific response of the body to any demand at a certain point in time, the general adaptation syndrome (G.A.S.) is Selye's concept which allows him to add the dimension of time to stress.[1] The G.A.S. includes all nonspecific changes as they develop throughout prolonged stress.

It has three characteristic stages (see Figure 6), the first of which is the alarm reaction. During this stage the body manifests the changes that accompany the initial exposure to a stressor. There are signs of confusion, disorientation, and distortion of reality. Resistance is down, and a strong stressor—such as a severe burn—could bring death. If the stressor doesn't cause death, yet remains present, this stage is followed by the second stage, that of resistance. Resistance rises above the normal level as most of the signs characteristic of the alarm reaction have vanished. Signs of this stage include fatigue, anxiety, tenseness, and extreme irritability. These first two stages are very normal as we all go through them many times. Only by doing so do we adapt enough to face the demands of life. Yet severe, prolonged stress could lead to the final stage—exhaustion.

The third stage of exhaustion is the one that catches everyone at the end of life. Exhaustion does not have to lead to death, because it can be reversed if it doesn't totally permeate the body. Running may produce exhaustion in the legs and cardiovascular system, but after a

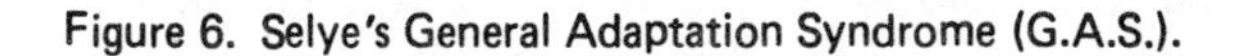

Figure 6. Selye's General Adaptation Syndrome (G.A.S.).

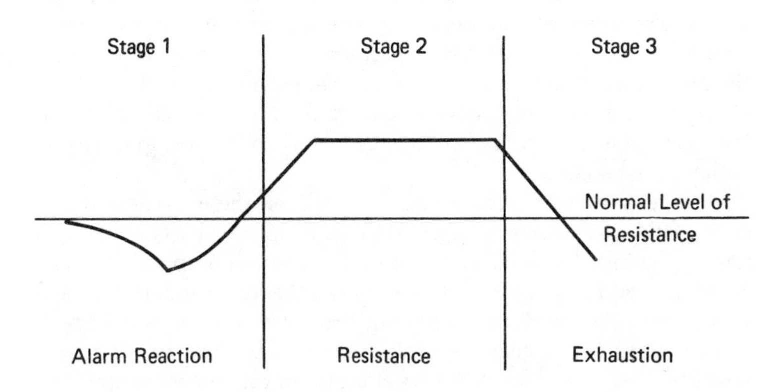

From the book *Stress Without Distress* by Hans Selye, M.D. Copyright © 1974 by Hans Selye, M.D. Reproduced by permission of J.B. Lippincott Company.

good rest we recover our strength. One of the signs of this stage is that there appears to be a point of no return at which apathy and emotional withdrawal set in.

The G.A.S. is different from the local adaptation syndrome (L.A.S.) in that it exists when several local adaptation syndromes are simultaneously working on you. The exhaustion of particular muscles would be an example of the last stage of an L.A.S. Most human activities go through a cycle much like the three stages of G.A.S.: you first have to get used to something new to get the swing of it; then you really get into it; finally, you tire and lose your interest and efficiency. These stages are also characteristic of an inflammation of the skin: A microbe getting under the skin first causes reddening, swelling, and pain (alarm reaction); then a chronic inflammation follows, such as the ripening of a boil (resistance); and finally the tissue's resistance is exhausted, allowing the boil to drain away its fluid (exhaustion).

The following work example shows the G.A.S. in action, although I have compressed the time span a bit for illustrative purposes. (Technically the G.A.S. does not work so quickly.) Suppose you come to work very early one day because you're excited about completing your budget before the day is over. You've been building yourself up psychologically for this day, and you think that you have all the data to complete the project by 5:00 that afternoon. By 9:00 A.M. you're sitting at your desk in a state of disorientation and confusion because so many unexpected problems have come up, threatening the possibility of your completing the budget that day. As you are sitting there wondering what else can go wrong, someone knocks on the door and informs you of another problem. You're now in stage one —the alarm reaction.

You resolve that you're not going to take all these problems lying down, and you decide to fight back with all the energy you can muster. Things continue to go badly for your game plan. It's now 10:45 A.M. and an old friend buzzes you on the intercom line and says very politely, "How about getting together for a nice long coffee break —we haven't had a chance to talk for a while." You respond with hostility: "Say, can't you leave me alone when you know I'm up to my ears in work? Am I the only one around here who puts out anymore?" You are now in the stage of resistance. You are very irritable, tense, anxious, and more tired than you should be by this time of day. (If this stress is prolonged for several days, you may experience the phenomenon of sleeping your usual number of hours each night but waking up still feeling fatigued. What happens is that you can't relax completely because your mind is vigorously working on your work problems.)

The final stage of exhaustion comes about 1:15 P.M. Things have continued to go poorly for you. You've not had a chance to go to lunch or even to take a break. Finally, your plans are dealt a devastating blow by some unexpected event, which finishes you off. You've reached a point of emotional apathy and withdrawal. You couldn't care less about completing your budget that day. Feelings of extreme fatigue and despair overwhelm you. If it's possible to leave the scene, you do so; if it's not possible to leave physically then you withdraw psychologically.

As indicated above, this example is slightly misleading because the time span of the events is accelerated. It's not uncommon, however, to see managers such as yourself in what amounts to a prolonged state of resistance—fighting back against various stressors that are affecting you adversely. You may discover that with time there are gradual changes in the normal "you." Prolonged resistance on your part, which is essentially an adaptive reaction, may change you so that being tense, irritable, anxious, and fatigued are now common for you, although they may have been uncommon in the past. I'm suggesting that when the characteristics of the resistance stage of the G.A.S. are persistent, these become danger signs and symptoms that you or your subordinates are under excessive stress for too long a time.

Selye indicates that although we can adapt remarkably well to adverse conditions such as are often found in the "dog eat dog" competitive climate of business, there are finite limits to the amount of adaptive energy we have. When the total amount allocated to us genetically is depleted, the signs of the alarm reaction reappear (Stage One), yet this time irreversibly so, thus bringing death. As Selye states:

> Our reserves of adaptation energy could be compared to an inherited fortune from which we can make withdrawals; but there is no proof that we can also make additional deposits. We can squander our adaptability recklessly, "burning the candle at both ends," or we can learn to make this valuable resource last long, by using it wisely and sparingly, only for the things that are worthwhile and cause least distress.[2]

Even though Selye freely admits that he can't prove this hypothesis, it is well worth taking heed of his speculations. You have probably noticed in yourself or in others how distress can age people rapidly. But the G.A.S. is only one method of gauging how well (or how poorly) people are handling stress; there are many signs and symptoms that can indicate when people are under excessive stress.

Danger signs at work

Busywork. One of the more innocuous signs of stress is a preoccupation with busywork. Sometimes when you face an unpleasant task, such as a boring report that you don't want to write, you may find yourself cleaning and straightening up your work area. Preoccupation with busywork functions at times almost as a security blanket for managers. Under the noble guise of "getting organized," you have a beautiful excuse to avoid distasteful chores.

Absenteeism. Excessive absenteeism among your subordinates may be a symptom of their being under too much pressure. Staying away from the source of stress is certainly one way to cope with stress, although absenteeism obviously isn't a long-range solution for anyone; it would be far better to confront the problem and deal with it directly. Absenteeism is a huge financial drain in both the private and public sectors. Certainly some of the absenteeism is caused by legitimate sickness, although much of it is due to lazy, irresponsible employees as well as to such chronic industry problems as alcoholism. However, it can't be denied that you or your subordinates may occasionally need to get away from the stressful situation or persons.

Defense Mechanisms. Defense mechanisms are a necessary and normal function of all human beings, yet some people develop a coping style that turns normal defense mechanisms into long-term, habitual defensiveness. Thus, one of several common defense mechanisms could become your primary way of dealing with stress. This chronic form of defensiveness is a health hazard because it allows you to avoid facing your situation realistically and taking constructive action either to eliminate the source of stress or to lessen its impact on you. Ask yourself if any of the defense mechanisms described below have become a regular part of your personality or of your subordinates' behavior.

Denial is a defensive behavior you use to avoid admitting that a problem exists. A sales manager who is under pressure from an aggressive competitor may handle it by saying, "I know our customers well. We've been good to them over the years, and they will be loyal to us even though our competitor is undercutting us in price." Or perhaps you've known a manager who was told by his peers and subordinates that his boss is unhappy with his performance. His boss also may have been hinting that some changes were needed. Yet despite these multiple messages, the manager says, "There's no problem. I know that top management still supports my work. Besides, if they tried to remove me, I would go to the board of directors. I have some good friends there who I know appreciate my work." In both of the above cases, the managers are using denial as an inadequate coping style.

Illusion is another common defense mechanism used by managers. A manager under pressure to cut costs and increase production in his department may say, "I'm doing all I can." Although this is rarely the case, he responds to the pressure by concocting an illusion. Of course, this defensive response prevents him from really looking carefully at how he might improve his department's performance.

Xenophobia, or the hatred of foreigners, is another defensive behavior you may see among managers. A frustrated sales manager under pressure to increase sales may say, "We're just not getting technically superior products from our research and development laboratory. If we were getting the right kind of products, our sales would be up considerably. But you can't sell inferior products." Or a manager in the field may remark, "If headquarters would quit making so many mistakes on the accounts of our customers, we wouldn't have them so upset with us, causing us to lose a number of them. We can't do our job well because those highly paid staff people at headquarters are always failing to give us the right kind of support."

Other defense mechanisms such as *rationalizations* could also be identified as inadequate coping styles developed on the foundation of defensive behavior which in its proper place is a necessary, normal behavioral pattern. Rationalization is the act of giving ostensibly logical excuses for misbehavior or disappointments. It isn't uncommon to hear a person who has been passed over for an important new position say, "I wouldn't take that job for anything. It requires far more travel than I'd be willing to do." We often end up believing our own rationalizations, although our friends know better.

Subpar Performance. One of the clearest warning signs of excessive stress among your subordinates is when they fall below their normal performance standards. When the criteria you use for judging performance are not being met by subordinates, you can rightly be suspicious that stress may be undermining an employee's ability to concentrate on his or her work.

If stress is the culprit and you don't recognize it, you may make matters worse by adding even more pressure to the situation, because if a person is already beyond his or her threshold and you add more stress, you'll most likely cause that person's performance to deteriorate even more rapidly. Discussing the poor work performance and the reasons for it is probably the only way to assess the situation fairly. This person may need emotional support and understanding, or he or she may be goofing off. You must get to the bottom of the matter. Be careful not to always assume that employees are under excessive stress when their performance is suddenly subpar—it may not be so. If your immediate response is to assume that stress is the culprit and you lighten the person's workload, you may find many other employees following suit, hoping for the same good deal from you. You may even get a reputation as a "soft touch." Yet a sudden drop in performance from one of your reliable employees should be given close scrutiny for the possibility that stress is involved. Of course, the danger sign could apply to your own work as well.

Rate of life changes

But, as I've pointed out before, there are many sources of stress *outside* work as well. Changes in normal life events, especially when those changes are severe, can disrupt our everyday behavioral patterns, induce stress, and even bring on illness. According to Drs. Thomas H. Holmes and Richard Rahe of the University of Washington School of Medicine, the rate of change in your life is related to the probability of a change in your health. You can adjust to only so many different life events in a period of time without encountering a high risk of illness or a health change of some kind. Holmes and Rahe developed the Social Readjustment Rating Scale, which ranks 43 life events according to the severity of adjustment that is necessitated by each of these events. Their severity is rated on a scale of zero to 100 Life Change Units (LCUs).[3] As you can see in Figure 7, taken from the above-mentioned study, the death of a spouse is thought to require twice as much adjustment as marriage. Being fired is twice as stressful as simply having trouble with the boss. Holmes and Rahe's findings are compatible with Selye's idea that pleasant stressors can be stressful and can require adaptation on your part. Marriage is normally a pleasant stressor, although few events in life require as much adjustment.

Note that any major change in your financial condition—whether you suddenly inherit a great amount of money or go bankrupt—carries with it 38 points. Item number 20, a mortgage over $10,000, should probably be interpreted as any large mortgage because in today's inflationary climate a mortgage as low as $10,000 is virtually unknown. An outstanding personal achievement has an adjustment

Figure 7. The social readjustment rating scale.

Life Event	Mean Value
1. Death of Spouse	100
2. Divorce	73
3. Marital separation	65
4. Jail term	63
5. Death of close family member	63
6. Personal injury or illness	53
7. Marriage	50
8. Fired at work	47
9. Marital reconciliation	45
10. Retirement	45
11. Change in health of family member	44
12. Pregnancy	40
13. Sex difficulties	39
14. Gain of new family member	39
15. Business readjustment	39
16. Change in financial state	38
17. Death of close friend	37
18. Change to different line of work	36
19. Change in number of arguments with spouse	35
20. Mortgage over $10,000	31
21. Foreclosure of mortgage or loan	30
22. Change in responsibilities at work	29
23. Son or daughter leaving home	29
24. Trouble with in-laws	29
25. Outstanding personal achievement	28
26. Wife begin or stop work	26
27. Begin or end school	26
28. Change in living conditions	25
29. Revision of personal habits	24
30. Trouble with boss	23
31. Change in work hours or conditions	20
32. Change in residence	20
33. Change in schools	20
34. Change in recreation	19
35. Change in church activities	19
36. Change in social activities	18
37. Mortgage or loan less than $10,000	17
38. Change in sleeping habits	16
39. Change in number of family get-togethers	15
40. Change in eating habits	15
41. Vacation	13
42. Christmas	12
43. Minor violations of the law	11

factor of 28 points. I'm sure you have known individuals who discovered that success brought the need for many adjustments in their lives.

A good example of this is boxer Leon Spinks, who was almost completely unknown when he won the world heavyweight championship from Muhammad Ali. (Ali won the title back seven months later.) Spinks's behavior—his spendthrift habits, his many traffic violations, his arrest for possession of marijuana and cocaine (the charges were later dropped)—is evidence of a man who was unprepared for so much success in so short a time and who was unable to make the adjustments that fame and prosperity demand. Success itself can be stressful, because once you're successful, everyone else (and perhaps you yourself) expect you to be at least as successful in the future as you have been in the past—if not more so.

A wife's beginning or stopping work creates the need for a lot of family adjustments, and normal family routines can be severely disrupted: A husband may suddenly find that the house is not as clean as it was before; dinner is later and not as scrumptious as before; shirts are not ironed in time; and many other routine chores that she used to do are left undone. In whatever way the family chooses to deal with this situation, you can be sure that everyone will have to make adjustments.

You may be surprised to find out that vacations and Christmas exact a toll, in stress, but consider what they are often like. You may save up many household chores as well as fun activities until your vacation time so that you end up cramming so much into your vacation period that you literally wear yourself out. A vacation is supposed to be refreshing and relaxing, yet you can turn it into two of the most hectic, fast-paced weeks of the year. Christmas is an exciting time of the year for almost everyone—there are parties, family gatherings with loved ones, shopping sprees, and a general excitement in the air—but in our efforts to get into the spirit of the season and enjoy ourselves, we sometimes push ourselves too far. As with our vacations, we can damage our health by squeezing too much activity into too short a time period.

You can calculate your own susceptibility to a health change in the near future by totaling the number of Life Change Units you have accumulated in the past year. If you have 150 or fewer points, you have a 33 percent chance of a serious health change in the next year (you already have a 10 percent chance of visiting a hospital each year); your chances rise to 50 percent if you have 150–300 points; and if you accumulate over 300 points, just get ready because you have an 80–90 percent chance for illness. Of course, as has been repeatedly emphasized throughout the book, your being in a high-risk group means only that you are in a high risk group; it doesn't necessarily mean that you as an individual will have a serious health change.

One of the real problems is that "When sorrows come, they come not single spies, / But in battalions!" *Hamlet*, IV: v). Rarely do single life events occur in isolation; rather, they are usually interconnected so that one life event evokes other changes as well. For example, getting a divorce (73 points) usually also entails these changes: sex difficulties (39), change in financial state (38), change in living conditions (25), revision of personal habits (24), change in residence (20), change in social activities (18), and a change in eating habits (15). You can imagine how high the total of LCUs could be if there were any other changes occurring in your life at the same time. During an especially heavy period of change and adjustment in your life, it might make good sense not to compound the problem by initiating additional changes over which you do have some control. For example, if you are undergoing a divorce, think twice before also quitting your job and going into business for yourself—especially if you're on vacation at Christmas time!

Changes in your life are not necessarily to be avoided: The very nature of human growth and development requires changes at various stages of life. Of course, not all changes are for the better, but many changes are. Yet the Holmes and Rahe research clearly indicates that too much change in too short a period of time exacts its toll on the body's adaptive capabilities, thus raising the risk of major health problems.

At this point a cautionary note from Selye is appropriate. There are a number of questionnaires available today to help you detect how much stress you're under. There are also some mechanical instruments that measure a few indicators of stress. Selye's reservation about all these attempts to measure stress is that none of these approaches, including that of Holmes and Rahe, makes any allowance for the significant difference between eustress and distress. Furthermore, these approaches also neglect this all-important fact: "It is our ability to cope with the demands made by the events in our lives, not the quality or intensity of the events, that counts."[1] Thus, we come back to the observation that how you take it is by far the most important determinant of whether intense stress is essentially good for you (eustress) or bad for you (distress).

Questionnaires, checklists, and instruments have their place, but you must be careful to use them wisely. The more different kinds of stress indicators you use, the more accurate your overall stress profile should be. So feel free to use the questionnaires and checklists in this book, but remember that none of these methods can capture a complete profile of you and your own unique responses to the stressors of life.

Danger signs and symptoms of stress

Selye believes that when you are "under stress" you tend to respond with a particular set of danger signs and symptoms that are caused by malfunctioning of the most vulnerable parts of your body. The weakest parts of your body may be the strongest parts of another's. You may have a tendency to get migraine headaches and an upset stomach, whereas someone else may experience pounding of the heart and pain in the lower back. Selye pinpoints 31 signs of danger that are easy enough for you to detect.[1] As you read his list of signs, think about which set of signs is characteristic of you "under stress."

1. General irritability, hyperexcitation, or depression
2. Pounding of the heart, an indicator of high blood pressure
3. Dryness of the throat and mouth
4. Impulsive behavior, emotional instability
5. The overpowering urge to cry or to run and hide
6. Inability to concentrate, flight of thoughts, and general disorientation
7. Feelings of unreality, weakness, or dizziness
8. Predilection to become fatigued, and loss of the "joie de vivre"
9. "Floating anxiety"—that is to say, we are afraid, although we do not know exactly what we are afraid of

10. Emotional tension and alertness, feeling of being "keyed up"
11. Trembling, nervous tics
12. Tendency to be easily startled by small sounds
13. High-pitched, nervous laughter
14. Stuttering and other speech difficulties
15. Bruxism, or grinding of the teeth
16. Insomnia
17. Hypermotility
18. Sweating
19. The frequent need to urinate
20. Diarrhea, indigestion, queasiness in the stomach, and sometimes even vomiting
21. Migraine headaches
22. Premenstrual tension or missed menstrual cycles
23. Pain in the neck or lower back
24. Loss of appetite or compulsive eating
25. Increased smoking
26. Increased use of legally prescribed drugs, such as tranquilizers or amphetamines.
27. Alcohol and drug addiction
28. Nightmares
29. Neurotic behavior
30. Psychoses
31. Proneness to accidents

Depression. Depression and anxiety are two of the most common signs of stress. Depression simply means a chronic, low-key sense of dejection about one's total situation in life. It is characterized by sadness, inactivity, lack of energy, and difficulty in sustaining mental concentration. This moodiness and lack of interest in life make it hard for the depressed person to perform even the most simple, everyday activities—much less the more complex functions of modern life.

Obviously some depression in response to tragic events in life, such as an unexpected death of someone close to you, is quite normal. But the form of depression to which I'm referring is a more generalized response—sometimes without any apparent cause. This form of depression is often susceptible to drug treatment, although there are probably better long-term solutions. I will discuss some of these later.

In general, depression is usually the result of some deficit in your life.[4] To overcome it you must replace what you have lost. One of the most common signs of depression to watch for is the tendency to overeat. A satisfied stomach seems to make us feel better. However, for some people just the opposite is true. When depressed, some lose their appetite. A change in sleep patterns (such as chronic oversleeping or waking up in the middle of the night for no apparent reason) is another indicator of depression. The sudden appearance of aches and pains is another tip-off that you may be depressed. According to Dr. Bertram S. Brown, the Director of the National Institute of Mental Health in 1974, some studies indicate that perhaps as many as 15 percent of the American adult population may suffer from serious symptoms of depression.

Anxiety. Anxiety is a pervasive, almost physical feeling of apprehension, dread, and "uptightness." But it is important to distinguish first between anxiety and fear, and second between anxiety and frustration. Fear is the reaction to specific, immediate danger; anxiety is the reaction to *anticipated* danger, the particular form of which may be unknown. People are frustrated when they are blocked from reaching their goals; people get anxious when they feel they don't have effective plans for dealing with the anticipated danger.

The core of most anxiety is personal worry about the many things that could go wrong: financial success or failure, career development, children, possible illness—almost anything. Other job-related matters that can provoke anxiety include instability because of frequent administrative changes, a volatile economic environment, competition, job ambiguity, lack of feedback about one's performance, and social isolation from one's colleagues. But regardless of its source, anxiety is a symptom of stress.

Insomnia. Insomnia plagues millions of Americans every year, and most people have suffered from it at some point in their lives. Whether it means waking up in the middle of the night or simply not being able to fall asleep, it is very draining on a person's energy level. Almost nothing is more frustrating than feeling a desperate need to go back to sleep and not being able to do so. The harder you try, the more awake you become. Of course, the reason you're suffering from insomnia is because you are excited (eustress) or anxious (distress) about the next day's events. Here again we see that pleasant stressors can be as stressful as unpleasant stressors. Chronic insomnia is a danger sign that you really are under too much stress, although to occasionally miss a night or two of sleep is a rather normal occurrence for most people. It probably does suggest the presence of some stress, but when the stress is eliminated, the insomnia also vanishes. Yet chronic insomnia due to constant stress spells trouble unless you take some action.

The American public usually attacks the problem of insomnia with a pill or a drink. Provided your physician approves, the occasional use of either of these remedies (but *never* both at the same time!) is not always bad, especially when you are truly facing intense stressors, such as adjusting to the death of a spouse. However, by far the best way to handle insomnia is to get your work done during the day or at least to get yourself organized with a game plan for how to attack your problems. Sometimes knowing how and when you are going to deal with certain problems will help set your mind at ease. One simple solution is to stay late at the office in order to solve some problem that will otherwise keep you awake all night. Staying at work a half hour or even an hour more is preferable to spending several sleepless, restless hours agonizing over what you didn't get done and worrying when you're going to do it.

Pain in Back or Neck. The symptoms of pain in the neck or lower back often are caused by your unknowingly tensing these muscles when you're in a stressful situation (see Chapter 1). When these muscles are chronically contracted, they are bound to become painful. So the expression about one who is creating stress—"He's a pain in the neck"—is sometimes literally true as well as being a colorful figure of speech.

Appetite. Regarding your appetite under stress, you may respond by overeating, whereas someone else may tend to undereat. Overeating can be a way of diverting attention from stressors and toward food. Physiologically, a full stomach and intestine use a great deal of blood. This increased demand for blood in the abdomen brings about a slight tranquilizing effect as a result of a slight decrease in blood circulating in the brain. Thus mental alertness is somewhat reduced. However, other people under stress experience stomach disorders which cause a decline in their appetite and eventual loss of weight. So gaining or losing weight could be an indication that you're under excessive stress and that the needle on your stress guage is too high.

Increased Smoking. An increase in the number of cigarettes you smoke is often a sign that you're experiencing more than your normal amount of stress. Psychologically, I'm told by smokers that when they're under stress some relief comes with the very first puff. Yet physiologically nicotine acts first as a stimulant and only later as a depressant. Nicotine does immediately increase your heart rate. (Check your pulse before and after smoking—the change should be noticeable.) Nicotine also acts on the body to temporarily raise blood pressure and levels of cholesterol and noradrenaline, a close relative of adrenaline. So, in effect, as Selye defines stress, the more nicotine you take into your system, the more stressed you will be. Of course, the basic point here regarding smoking is that increased smoking is very likely a meaningful danger sign of stress for smokers.

Increased Drinking. An increase in your consumption of alcoholic beverages is another symptom of excessive stress. The real problem with alcohol as a stress reliever is that it works so well in causing you to forget the source of your discomfort and to focus on the "eustress of psychic elation, or at least tranquilization."[1] Because it does bring your system down and allow you to relax, you may begin to drink more and more. If you're not careful, you may soon have a severe drinking problem and be looking to the bottle for the solution to the problems that are causing your stress.

Alcoholism is a serious problem in industry precisely because it does initially help you get away from it all, although the judicious use of alcohol is probably safer and better than taking pills regularly. Usually a social drinker becomes a problem drinker as he or she begins to encounter more and more pressure at work or at home. Thus, by monitoring the amount that you drink, you can detect when early warning signs of distress appear. If you suspect that you may be an alcoholic, answer the following questions from the test for an alcoholic devised by Dr. Harry Johnson when he was chairman of the Medical Board of the Life Extension Institute.[5]

1. Do you drink six or more ounces of whisky a day?
2. Do you always have a couple of cocktails at lunch even when alone?
3. Do you stop for a quick drink at night on the way home from work?

4. Do you habitually order "doubles" when you drink?
5. Do you sometimes "forget" to eat after you've had a few drinks?
6. Do you often sneak drinks in the kitchen?
7. Do you start drinking in the morning on weekends?

If you find that you have given more "yes" than "no" answers to these questions, you should seek medical attention.

Increased Caffeine Intake. Excessive intake of caffeine may be a danger sign of stress as well as an additional physiological stressor on your system. It is rather common to see coffee drinkers increase their consumption when they're under stress. The average cup of coffee contains 100–150 mg of caffeine. Nervousness, insomnia, headaches, sweaty palms, and perhaps ulcers have all been related to as little as 250 mg of caffeine. People who drink as few as three cups of coffee may develop the above conditions. Excessive amounts of caffeine can cause you to exhibit the same clinical signs as people suffering from anxiety. You have probably experienced that "edgy" feeling so common after heavy doses of caffeine.

Reliance upon sleeping pills, aspirin, or even laxatives may also be an indication of distress at work. These escapist methods don't allow you to get at the underlying causes of distress, and sometimes actually contribute more stress.

Disease: the ultimate result

In the conceptual model of stress which we are using (see Chapter 3), you will recall that various stressors at work and various extra-organizational stressors impinge upon you at the same time. Your own individual make-up determines how you will respond to these stressors. To the extent that you find yourself in distress, you begin to exhibit certain danger signs and symptoms that are most likely to be a distinct set of signs which are uniquely yours. If you don't heed these warning signs, you'll have a much greater chance of getting a disease —either coronary artery disease, psychosomatic illness, a mental health disorder, or other disease.

According to Kenneth R. Pelletier, standard medical textbooks indicate that 50 to 80 percent of all disease is psychosomatic or stress-related in origin. (In Chapter 1 we discussed a number of these diseases.) Some of these are peptic ulcers, ulcerative colitis, bronchial asthma, hay fever, arthritis, hypertension, hyperthyroidism, irregular heartbeat, migraine headaches, impotence, general sexual dysfunctions, sleep-onset insomnia, alcoholism, and the whole range of neurotic and psychotic disorders. If you begin to experience early signs of these diseases and take preventive action in time, you can perhaps avoid the fully developed disease, or at least minimize its impact and duration.

A SPECIAL CASE: SEXUAL DYSFUNCTION

Sexual dysfunction has been discussed very frequently of late, and its incidence is high. But what is often overlooked is that sexual dysfunction is both an initiator and a consequence of stress. Unfortunately, "sex is an early victim of stress," and "poor sex or no sex builds stress and there is nothing easier than to let that stress feed on itself and grow."[6] If you happen to have a single experience with impotence due to stressful conditions at the time, you may end up creating additional incidents of impotence by worrying about it unduly. It is a self-fulfilling prophecy: Based on your one bad experience, you begin to worry about failing the next time around, and your worrying brings on the very failure you so desperately wanted to avoid; it becomes a vicious circle. If you could perform sexually, your anxiety about it would vanish, but your anxiety spoils your capability to perform effectively. Hence, you are caught in your own trap until you can free yourself by trusting yourself to be able to complete the sexual act.

Human beings need healthy sex lives because sexual release is one of the most natural methods for alleviating stress. (More will be said about sex as a natural stress reduction technique in Chapter 5.) The point here is that distress may lead you to neglect sex or to have trouble with it just when you need it the most. The consequences of not having sexual satisfaction are well known (short temper, irritability, and an inability to concentrate well), and sexual dysfunctions are very frequently related to heavy stress in your own life or in the relationship between you and your partner. When the relationship between two people is going well and is not laden with stress, the sexual life of the two is usually very fulfilling.

The physical and mental signs of stress—two checklists

The following two checklists[6] are not precise enough to provide an accurate assessment of you, but they can be a beginning point for reflection. If you have more than two of these physical signs, you may be placing your body under high risk from excessive stress.

Physical Signs

1. Excess weight for your age and height
2. High blood pressure
3. Lack of appetite
4. A desire to eat as soon as a problem arises
5. Frequent heartburn
6. Chronic diarrhea or constipation
7. An inability to sleep
8. A feeling of constant fatigue
9. Frequent headaches
10. A need for aspirin or some other medication daily
11. Muscle spasms
12. A feeling of fullness although you've not eaten
13. Shortness of breath
14. A liability to fainting or nausea
15. An inability to cry or a tendency to burst into tears easily
16. Persistent sexual problems (frigidity, impotence, fear)
17. Excessive nervous energy which prevents sitting still and relaxing.

More than four of the following mental symptoms (or a total of four physical and mental symptoms) also indicate you're a high risk candidate from excessive stress.

Mental Signs

1. A constant feeling of uneasiness
2. Constant irritability with family and work associates
3. Boredom with life
4. A recurring feeling of being unable to cope with life
5. Anxiety about money
6. Morbid fear of disease, especially cancer and heart disease

7. Fear of death—your own and others'
8. A sense of suppressed anger
9. An inability to have a good laugh
10. A feeling of being rejected by your family
11. A sense of despair at being an unsuccessful parent
12. Dread as the weekend approaches
13. Reluctance to take a vacation
14. A feeling you can't discuss your problems with anyone
15. An inability to concentrate for any length of time or to finish one job before beginning another one
16. A terror of heights, enclosed spaces, thunderstorms, or earthquakes

Remember that the appropriate response to this entire chapter on danger signs and symptoms of stress is not blind panic, but awareness. This chapter should provide a basis for your becoming aware of to what extent you, and perhaps your subordinates, are pressing beyond the stress threshold or the elastic limits. These danger signs serve as red flags or circuit breakers to warn us when we are headed down the path toward disease. But once we are aware, the next step is to seek appropriate solutions, and it is to that task we turn in the next two chapters.

REFERENCES

1. Hans Selye, *The Stress of Life* (New York: McGraw-Hill, 1976).
2. Hans Selye, *Stress Without Distress* (New York: Signet, 1974).
3. Thomas H. Holmes and T. Stephenson Holmes, "How Change can Make Us Ill," *Stress* (Chicago: Blue Cross Association, 1974).
4. Sidney Lecker, *The Natural Way to Stress Control* (New York: Grosset and Dunlap, 1978).
5. Harry J. Johnson, *Executive Life-Styles: A Life Extension Institute Report on Alcohol, Sex and Health* (New York: Thomas Y. Crowell Company, 1974).
6. Jack Tresidder (ed.), *Feel Younger, Live Longer* (Chicago: Rand McNally, 1977).

CHAPTER 5

Stress-Reduction Insights

As I have emphasized throughout this book, you may sometimes need to increase the amount of stress in your life because your life has become flat and sterile; at other times, you may need to reduce stress because it's excessive and is becoming distressful. These approaches should also be used by you in your management of others: At times, you may need to become a stressor for others to increase their productivity; at other times, you may need to help others reduce excessive stress because it's making them ineffective and unproductive.

The basic options

Before proceeding any further, we must establish a broader viewpoint of stress management. When you are experiencing a strong stressor or perhaps several stressors, you have three basic options open to you: (1) tolerate the enemy, (2) fight back, or (3) retreat.

The analogy to the workings of the body is uncanny. It has been demonstrated that the body's homeostasis (the tendency of the body to maintain biochemical equilibrium or a steady state) depends upon two reactions, syntoxic and catatoxic. Syntoxic reactions act as tranquilizers, allowing a state of mutual passive tolerance between the body and the aggressor. Catatoxic reactions create chemical changes in which enzymes attack the aggressor and engage it in a death struggle. Cortisone is one of the best known syntoxic hormones. One of several anti-inflammatory corticoids (hormones of the adrenal cortex), cortisone inhibits inflammation and many defensive immune reactions of the body. Inhibiting inflammation is desirable when an innocuous foreign agent (an allergen such as pollen) incites the inflammation—for example, of the nose and eyes as in hay fever. Suppressing the defensive inflammation is the cure. Yet, when the aggressor is truly dangerous, your body initiates defensive reactions by means of catatoxic substances which carry the message to your tissues that an all-out war is required. Unfortunately, nature does not always know what is best: Sometimes your body reacts defensively, as in the case of an allergy attack, to a far greater extent than is required because the allergen is basically harmless. This overreaction creates the phenomenon of hay fever.

Selye gives the following example to illustrate how your reactions to a personal or organizational stressor parallel those reactions of your own body: You're walking down the street when a helpless drunk confronts you and begins insulting you. It's clear that he can't do any harm to you, and if you take a "syntoxic" attitude and ignore him, nothing will probably come of it. However, if you take a "catatoxic" attitude and prepare to fight him or actually do start a fight, you may cause yourself damage by getting worked up even if he doesn't hurt you. However, if the drunk is attacking you with a knife, a catatoxic response might be your only proper response—if it's too late to flee. As Selye puts it, "Both on the cellular and interpersonal level, we do not always recognize what is and what is not worth fighting."[1]

The point is that as you face stressors in life, you have the same approaches available to you as your body does when it's fighting a disease-causing agent. Actually you have one possibility that your body lacks—you can sometimes get away from the stressor; your body has only the catatoxic and syntoxic choices. In the real world, it's important to assess carefully which of these three approaches is likely to provide the greatest payoff in any given situation. Sometimes a wrong choice could be literally fatal.

Suppose you have a boss for whom you hate to work. He's mean, insensitive, unrealistic in his demands, and to top it all, incompetent. You may decide to react catatoxically by waging a political fight to wrest from him his position of power over you, although you should decide on this approach only after carefully assessing your chances of success, because if you miscalculate, it will be political suicide for you.

Or let's suppose that you opt for a syntoxic approach, trying to coexist peacefully by learning to put up with him because you're getting your satisfaction in life outside work. Such an approach may work, but a miscalculation could result in your suffering even more than before. For example, because of your efforts to "stomach" your boss and his abuse, you could end up with a bleeding ulcer in a few years. Or you may find that his behavior upsets you so much that your outside activities are adversely affected.

Your other option would be to get away from this tyrant by transferring to another department or by leaving the company entirely. Sometimes a flight response is best; sometimes it isn't. Taking such a response too quickly could lead to a pattern of avoiding unpleasant situations rather than dealing directly with them. If neither a catatoxic nor a syntoxic response appears appropriate, flight may indeed be your best tactic.

The stress-reduction insights and techniques described in this chapter and in the following one include all three of the above approaches. Most of the techniques are syntoxic, enabling you to put up with stressors in your life because of the compensating nature of those techniques. The insights employ a mixture of the three approaches. Incidentally, the distinction made here between insights and techniques is derived from a slightly different emphasis: Insights are geared more toward understanding the problems and then taking appropriate action; techniques are more oriented toward finding practical methods.

Self-esteem improvement

Improving your own sense of self-esteem is an effective stress-reduction insight. You will recall from Chapter 2 that each of us has an individually determined range for coping well with stress. We called it your adaptive range or elastic limits. As long as your stress gauge shows that you're within your elastic limits, you won't be subject to distress, but once the needle on your stress gauge crosses your threshold point, you'll begin to experience the effects of distress.

Think of it this way: You have 100 points of adaptive energy or capability, and you can adapt satisfactorily to the various demands of life as long as they don't cause you to exceed 100 points, but your performance will begin to deteriorate the moment you reach 101 points. Now these 100 points are available to help you cope well with all the demands of life. If you think of the sources of the demands to which you have to respond and adapt, you will see that three areas tend to dominate—work, family and social life, and your own self-concept. Of course, all three areas are interrelated, and the demands from one area tend to spill over into the others. We can't neatly compartmentalize our lives. It also stands to reason that if you are spending 30 of your available 100 points of adaptive energy on the demands in one area, then you will have only 70 points left for all the other demands of life to which you must respond.

Your self-concept is probably the most important area, because it is always with you, and you probably have the potential for controlling it more than any other area of your life. If your own self-concept is consuming 30 points and you can reduce that number to 10 points, you will have automatically increased by 20 points the amount of adaptive energy you can apply to the other areas of your life.

Improvement in self-esteem is no small task. William Glasser identifies two basic psychological needs that are closely related to how you feel about yourself: (1) the need to love and be loved, and (2) the need to feel worthwhile to yourself and others.[2] When these two essential psychological needs are met, you are not likely to suffer unduly from an inadequate or low self-concept. Erich Fromm supports Glasser by saying that optimal fulfillment in life is possible to you only if you have a truly intimate love relationship with at least one other person.[3] He isn't necessarily speaking of sexual intimacy, but rather of a relationship which is mutually nourishing to both partners and which of course would include sexual intimacy. Certainly, many people would agree that giving and receiving love provides some of the most marvelous peak experiences available to anyone.

The second need cannot be met simply by *thinking* about being worthwhile to ourselves and others; to feel worthwhile, you have to *do* something that justifies this feeling. All the world's great religions address these two psychological needs by teaching that you will truly find yourself only by submerging your own ego in service to another or to some worthy cause. Happiness with yourself comes as a by-product when you are reaching out to something greater, or to something or someone other than yourself.

Erik Erikson, whose theory of the eight stages of psychosocial development provides a theoretical basis for understanding the midlife crisis, indicates that in the middle years of life human beings have a need to be needed.[4] Healthy psychological development requires you to at least have the opportunity to be generative, or to exercise a parental concern over something—be it your work, your children, your garden, or anything else—during this period of your life. Those who fail to be generative because they haven't produced anything over which they can exercise guidance, often end up in a state of stagnation in which they tend to become their own parents and to exert parental concern over themselves, thereby degenerating into a state of self-absorption. Paradoxically, we often feel best about ourselves when we are not focusing upon ourselves; it is in giving that we find a self that is worthwhile to ourselves and others.

Stability zones

As was noted in Chapter 4, Holmes and Rahe show that too many changes in life events over too short a period of time can literally make us ill. We live in a changing, turbulent world in which adapting to the various changes is stressful. Therefore, establishing "stability zones" can help reduce the amount of stress you must cope with. A stability zone is an area of your life in which little or no change is taking place, or is occurring at a relatively slower pace than in other areas of your life. By maintaining high stability in some areas of your life, you can reserve a substantial amount of adaptive capabilities for other areas of your life which are changing more rapidly. Stability zones serve as anchors or moorings for your life.

For some people, religion may provide a source of stability. Religion often has an integrating, centering impact on an individual's life, helping to put things in perspective and to order one's priorities. Close family ties may also serve as a stability zone. Customs and family traditions help to provide a sense of security in the midst of so much insecurity in the world. Engaging in the same line of work for many years, or perhaps even working for the same company for a long period of time, are other examples of sources of stability. Living in the same neighborhood or the same house, keeping the same close friends for a long period of time, or perhaps even having certain material possessions may provide some sense of stability for people.

Interestingly enough, routine and rituals help to provide a stabilizing factor in people's lives. Can you imagine what life would be like if there were no routine? The next time you get upset with routine activites, imagine how you would feel if every waking moment presented a completely new, unexpected experience; such a situation would drive most of us "up the wall" within a few hours. The point here is simple, yet important: If you already have several sources of stability in your life, hang onto them tenaciously and make sure that they continue to serve you well. And as you contemplate your own situation, if you discover that stability zones are few and far between, you might consider trying to add more of them to your life.

Practicing good management

Oddly enough, practicing good management is one stress-reduction insight which when acted upon can be very effective. Being an effective and efficient manager will surely keep you enough on top of your work so that the stress load will be manageable. What I have in mind here in particular is that some managers go through their entire careers covering or hiding weaknesses that they are afraid to reveal to others. If you are deficient in certain managerial skills that you regularly have to use, don't go through the rest of your life being under stress every time you have to use that particular skill; try to master that skill as much as you can so that it does not create a sense of dread and terror and stress every time you have to exercise it. Every manager has weaknesses and inadequacies. If your particular skill proficiency is in an area which you almost never have to exercise, then perhaps it won't be worthwhile to spend the necessary time, money, and energy upgrading yourself.

For example, if in your job you regularly have to make formal, public presentations to audiences consisting of clients, colleagues, government officials, or just the general public, and such presentations create high levels of stress for you, then you really should consider taking a course in presentations or perhaps watching yourself on a videotape recorder, playing it back, and learning to improve your skills. Whatever the methods, you can't afford to live with this stress on a regular basis, especially if presentations are an important part of what you have to do to be effective.

Or to take another example, perhaps you have never learned how to delegate properly. Perhaps the whole process has always seemed very confusing to you, and you have always thought delegating authority meant abdication of responsibility and loss of control. You may need to take a seminar in delegation, talk to managers who do delegate effectively without seeming to lose control, and understand and learn the process of delegation. By doing so, you will eliminate one source of stress in your managerial life, and gain new confidence in your newly found skill. The payoff is well worth the effort.

Or perhaps you haven't learned to manage your time well. Effective time management is a key ingredient in a successful manager's repertoire of skills. Here again there are plenty of good courses and people who should be able to help in improving this particular skill. In fact, learning to delegate is one of the very best ways to improve the amount of discretionary time you have for your own concerns. These examples all illustrate the basic point: Whatever skill deficiency is serving as a source of stress for you, if you are regularly called upon to exercise this skill, then become proficient in it—and the stress will disappear.

Improving qualifications

Strengthening your personal and professional qualifications by keeping them as impeccable as possible is another good way to reduce stress. If you are an underutilized, undercompensated, or underappreciated person, you have basically three options: (1) You can try to get your management to see you differently—that is, you can encourage them to use you better, pay you better, and appreciate you more. (Perhaps a dramatic display of your value to management will pay off.) (2) You can work for a transfer within your present company. (3) You can leave your company and find a less stressful job. The person with the strongest qualifications has the best chance of making any one of these three options work, and believing that you do have options can help you decide whether to put up with the stress you are facing. This is one good reason for actually *market-testing* your options, as the following true story illustrates.

A middle-aged engineer with a large aerospace firm had been asking his management for a long time to change his assignment because he was tired of it, but his bosses had ignored him. One day, this man, who had worked for this company for more than 20 years, cleaned out his desk and suddenly quit his job. His superiors were shocked—they had never believed that he would take such a drastic step. This man did not look for another job, yet the word got out in the aerospace industry that he was available. He was a man who had kept his qualifications impeccable and within two days, without his seeking it, he had two solid, excellent offers from competing firms.

Eventually the man decided to return to his original company, but only because other people at the company offered him a better assignment. But he came back a different man, freely choosing to put up with the stress that was connected with his new job and knowing full well that if things did not go his way at any moment, he could go elsewhere. He not only believed he had options in the marketplace; he *knew* it, because he had *market-tested* it. The confidence that such a market test provides cannot be overestimated, so if you keep your qualifications as strong as possible and if you know that you have options, then you will be in a better position to deal with the stress that comes your way. Try never to be in a position where you feel you have no options, because this will only compound any stress that you are facing and will increase the likelihood that a great deal of stress can become distressful for you.

Good mental health

Another good stress-reduction insight is to develop and practice good mental-health habits. A strong psychological adjustment on the part of an individual is known to effectively help offset the dysfunctional effects of stress. Back in the 1950s Lawrence Shaffer and Edward Shoben, Jr., formulated a list of conditions for good mental health which have withstood the test of time. These good mental-health habits or practices, although obviously not the only ones, are a good representative list.[5]

1. *Good physical health* increases your resistance to physical and psychological stressors. Today the general public and the medical world are keenly aware of the vital connection between the mind and the body. Healthy bodies breed healthy minds; unhealthy bodies eventually breed unhealthy minds. And the converse is also true: Healthy minds breed healthy bodies; unhealthy minds tend to breed unhealthy bodies. More and more physicians are coming to endorse this statement—a growing number of them believe that fully 50–80 percent of all illness is psychosomatic in origin. A strong, well-conditioned body is more resilient in the face of both physical and psychological stressors.

2. *Accept yourself.* Accepting yourself for who you are with all of your strengths, weaknesses, failures, and successes is indeed part of good mental health. Realistic self-acceptance excludes smug complacency and phoniness. Acceptance of the realities about yourself is a continual process throughout life; it is never "over and done with." Self-acceptance is not an easy task, but it is an essential one.

In our society, where self-improvement is a national preoccupation (and a multimillion-dollar industry), people latch on to various techniques that promise increased self-knowledge but often have negative effects on our behavior. For example, although I am skeptical of some of the claims that have been made for the importance of biorhythms, I feel that biorhythms can help explain the ebb and flow of moods, emotions, and mental abilities, which we all experience from day to day. However, some people attribute every personal disaster to the effects of biorhythms; or if they discover that their biorhythm chart indicates they will be emotionally unstable that day, they may act in such a way as to confirm that prognosis, thereby turning simple information about biorhythms into a self-fulfilling prophecy.

I believe that anybody can overcome the depressed feelings that may result from certain biorhythms and can cope with the problems of daily life even on days when our biorhythm charts show that we are at our lowest. Self-acceptance certainly involves acceptance of *all* our moods—be they euphoric or depressed; be they caused by biology or by the circumstances of our lives. But accepting the existence of these different moods does not mean that you cannot counteract some of their more deleterious effects.

3. *Maintaining a confidante,* or someone with whom you can talk with the utmost trust, is another stress-reduction insight. If this confidante happens to be a spouse, it makes for great communication in marriage, but if for some reason or another you are not able to confide in a spouse (or if you don't have one), you do need someone with whom you can share your feelings. Telling someone else what's bothering you can play a vital role in combating tension. It is not at all uncommon for consultants to act as confidantes for top management by serving as sounding boards and as sympathetic listeners. When people in top management have nobody else on whom they can unload what is on their minds, they would be well advised to use consultants for that purpose.

4. *Taking constructive action to eliminate the source of the stress* is another good mental health practice. If you are an underutilized, undercompensated, and underappreciated engineer, you can get only so far in talking about that with a confidante. It certainly helps to talk, but good mental health also calls for constructive action. You may have to make a dramatic show of worth in order to get your management to pay you better, appreciate you more, and use you more to your own liking.

5. *Interacting with people with whom you don't work.* Sometimes this problem exists in large organizations, but most of the time it happens in small organizations. It is not particularly healthy to socialize exclusively with people with whom you work daily, because you may have the tendency to keep talking shop even while you are socializing. Your social life should provide at least some opportunity to get away from the complaints and problems that you face daily at work. Selye himself has strongly suggested that stress can be equalized by the principle of deviation or shifting work from one point to another. In fact he puts it this way: "The human body—like the tires on a car or the rug on a floor—wears longest when it wears evenly."[6] Certainly it is all right to have friends, even close friends, among your coworkers, but you may be ignoring the important principle of deviation in your life if you associate exclusively with work peers.

6. *Creative experiences promote mental health.* These creative ex-

periences may occur within your vocation or avocation, and in either case they can be a very healthy change from the kind of thinking that you are normally used to. For example, one top manager I know has recently started the practice of flying to San Francisco and then bicycling down the Pacific Coast Highway from San Francisco to Los Angeles, taking one week to complete the route. He finds the experience extremely refreshing, creative, and invigorating. His job requires a fair amount of conceptual work as well as paperwork, and he comes back from his week's vacation with a clear mind.

Hobbies are a great example of creative experiences that refresh you. Using the principle of deviation, hobbies or creative experiences bring a change of pace and relaxation to your life. The important thing here is to have some hobby that works for you and, as you probably know, what works for other people may not work as a creative hobby for you. Gardening drives some people crazy, although for others it can be a relaxing antidote to boredom. Being a handy person around the house is relaxing for some and extremely stressful for others.

7. *Do meaningful work.* If you have a job that you thoroughly enjoy, then think very carefully about giving it up even if a new job means a few more dollars and higher status. In my most idealistic moments I sometimes wonder what the world would be like if everyone had a job that was meaningful and enjoyable. I know what it would be like—it would be paradise on earth, because there would be no internal tension, no national tension, and very few family pressures; everyone would feel useful and fulfilled. Most people in the world don't have the opportunity to have meaningful jobs, although managers and professional people in general have a much better chance of working themselves into such a position. Don't underestimate the value of having a job you truly enjoy.

While driving on a freeway in Los Angeles in 1977, I heard an interview with the well-known newscaster Paul Harvey who was celebrating his twentieth anniversary on radio. Among the things he said, one particular comment stood out: "I probably shouldn't say this on the radio, because management may be listening, but I honestly enjoy my work so much that I believe I would have done it for the past 20 years if management had not paid me a dime. In fact, I can't think of any other job in the whole world that I would rather do than what I do every day of the week. I don't consider my job work; it's play!"

Selye himself suggests that having a job that you consider to be play rather than work is one of the best ways of reducing stress. It is also going to be conducive to good mental health. If you have a job that is enjoyable to you, then even though there are stressors associated with that job—as inevitably there will be—those are stressors that you *enjoy* dealing with. They constitute eustress rather than distress. Rather than harming you, these stressors may *stimulate* you to a greater and more fruitful way of life.

8. *Use the scientific method on your personal problems.* If a manager is anything he is a problem solver. You probably use your analytical skills to solve problems daily in your work. However, many a manager fails to be able to use such skills when faced with emotionally laden personal problems, yet if he would bring the resources to bear upon these problems as well, he might find solutions that he wouldn't discover otherwise.

The single biggest problem in bringing the scientific method to bear on personal problems is that of *problem identification.* You may often solve a problem only to find that it's not the most important one. For example, perhaps you and your spouse are having sexual difficulties. The two of you sit down, analyze the situation, and decide that your problem is that neither one of you wants to sleep with the other—in short, your desire for one another is gone. You look at your alternatives and decide to go to a clinic for people who have sexual dysfunctions. If the clinic is indeed a good one, it may help you to discover that you didn't have a sexual problem but a problem in your relationship: You had stopped communicating deeply with each other about your feelings.

In this particular example, you can see how failing to adequately identify the problem only hindered your ability to find the appropriate answer. Don't assume that you can't be analytic and scientific in both identifying problems and seeking their solution in your personal life. You can do so if you are willing to try. Easy it may not be, but it *is* possible.

Cognitive strategies

Both external and internal stressors are filtered through the individual's personality, and that personality determines how strong the stress reaction will be: Some individuals can take the sting out of a rather powerful stressor; others are thrown by the mildest of stressors. It is the difference between being able to roll with the punch and not being able to do so, thereby taking the full force of the stressor without any cushioning.

One of the main factors in determining your reaction to stressors is the cognitive process of perception. How you perceive or think about a particular stressor is all important. Therefore managing your thoughts is an effective means of reducing or equalizing stress. To say that stress is all in your mind is too simplistic: Stress is not just in the mind, but your mental efforts can help you minimize stress. The following discussion will focus on some of these cognitive strategies.

First, don't revert to simplistic thinking; rather, make your thinking as complex as possible. With excessive stress, strong feelings of arousal—even agitation—usually appear. As you become more upset, your thoughts tend to revert to a more primitive, simplistic state. "Tunnel vision" sets in; and you become oblivious to your environment. More sophisticated and complex ways of coping with a situation give way to primitive simplification. Instead of reverting to simplistic thinking, you need to keep your mind alert to other ways of interpreting what's happening to you.

Karl E. Weick has provided an illustration of how this process might work when you are faced with an overload of input which is taxing your ability to respond intelligently.[7] Suppose that instead of saying, "I can't handle it," or getting ill or running away from the pressing demands, you decide to stay mentally alert and analyze what's going on. You decide to analyze each word in your statement, "I can't handle it."

Look at the first word, "I." Are you the only one who can't handle it, or would most others not be able to handle it, either? Can you give the problem to someone who can handle it? The second word, "can't," is also susceptible to further analysis. Are you sure you can't handle it, or is it that you don't want to deal with it, even though you're able to do so? Could you substitute "can try to" for "can't"? The simple statement, "I can't handle it," carries enough unpleasant implications to blind you to other possibilities; a more complex response may inhibit this blinding effect.

The word "handle" can also be looked at from a different perspective: Do you have to handle it perfectly? Finally, what precisely is "it"? Getting a clear definition of "it" may put the problems in a new light. A problem can be viewed from many different angles, and be careful not to let stress overload cause you to adopt a form of tunnel vision which will prevent you from seeing other, perhaps less stressful solutions to the problem.

Second, recognize that the stress will not last forever. When you're under tremendous stress, it's not uncommon to begin to think that it will never end. But if you have had enough experience, it will be helpful to recall that the acute stress of a certain time will diminish in magnitude and eventually vanish. You can also try to imagine what it will be like when the stressful situation is over. This method of thinking in the future perfect tense ("I shall have solved that problem") will help convince you that your current difficulties will end and may help you focus on ways of solving the problem so that you will be able to arrive at that point.

For example, let's say you're trying to decide whether to change jobs. You're under a great deal of stress because you want to do what's best professionally for your career and for your family as well. By imagining that the future has already happened and by envisioning what it will be like, you will see that the heavy stress will eventually subside. By examining what you think *might* happen, you may gain insights into what you really want to do now. Projecting an event as an accomplished fact usually facilitates its analysis.

Third, keep your head in the midst of unsettling stressors. W. Timothy Gallwey uses the term "freak-out" to describe an upset mind.[8] Even though it may well describe a tennis player's reaction to a poor shot, it applies equally well to other situations in life when your mind is so upset (stressed) that you can't think clearly about what action to take. Action based on freaked-out thinking isn't usually very appropriate or effective. For example, when you're under a lot of pressure and are not feeling well, you get a time sheet back from your payroll department indicating an extremely minor error. As you investigate the reason for it, you have to deal on the phone with a clerk in the payroll department who has an insulting, disrespectful manner. Being freaked out, you march over to see her and insult her and criticize her poorly written note. You end up complying with her request, but also trying to match her insult for insult. This whole incident would get you no where and would damage future relations with your payroll people.

Typically, the reasons for freak-outs can be classified into three categories: dislike of a present situation (as above), regret about past events, and fear or uncertainty about the future. Let's look at what may happen when regret about a past event upsets your mind. You hire a secretary who quickly makes a disaster area of your office. You fire her, but as you do, you think to yourself, "I must be a terrible interviewer and judge of people." Before long, you are really down on yourself as you analyze the situation: "She was terrible. I should have spotted her weaknesses in the interview. I am an atrocious judge of people. And because being a good judge of people is such an important quality in an effective manager, I must be a lousy manager." You are probably way off base in your analysis, because that's what frequently happens when you freak out. In this case you're letting one mistake represent far too much, and you're failing to see the positive side: you did fire her when you realized your mistake. For after all, the ability to rectify mistakes is also a characteristic that effective managers possess. Yet it's the nature of freaked-out thinking that you don't see the whole picture clearly in perspective.

Now let's see what may happen when you are fearful or uncertain about the future. To illustrate future "freak out," let's carry the above example further. Now you're about to interview prospective applicants to replace the secretary. As you are about to begin an interview, the following thoughts run through your mind: "What if I blow it again by making another poor choice? What will my boss and my own staff think? I just can't afford to make a mistake this time. I'll never hear the end of it." It should be rather evident that this kind of thinking is certainly not going to help you in your selection process. The answer is to see that the problem is more in your mind than in the external situation—it's your reaction that counts. By keeping your head and remaining calm you'll be able to find the resources for dealing with the situation successfully.

As strange as it may seem, there appears to be truth in the idea that just letting go and "letting it happen" often increases your effectiveness. When you give too much attention to details, your performance may be affected. I know it's true in tennis, and I believe it's true in the world of management as well. When I think mechanically and am constantly worried about technique, I fail to be as fluid and effective a player as I can be. After I have learned how to hit the ball, I must let go and let my body do what I've trained it to do. In management it's the same thing: You certainly may have to learn and practice the skills of management, but at a certain point of maturity you must let go and let your management style be—you must let it happen. Letting it happen is a process of trusting yourself, your experience, your training, and your natural responses. When you don't let it happen, you wind up being a stilted, rigid bureaucrat who passes as a manager. When you do let it happen, you wind up being a responsive, effective manager who has fully integrated his training, experiences, and unique personality. If you're that kind of manager, you'll trust your own potential and learn to rely on natural processes that turn your potential into actual results.

What some have called coping self-statements constitute a fourth way of using your head to combat excessive stress.[9] Coping self-statements are simply the words you say to yourself as you deal with a particular source of stress. It's the old-fashioned remedy of "talking to yourself"; the only difference is that you decide ahead of time what thoughts you're going to feed yourself in the midst of the stress. You want to be sure to speak thoughts to yourself that are going to enable you to cope better than you otherwise would. Obviously, you don't want to feed yourself ideas that will only increase the stress and hinder your coping mechanism.

There are four situations in which you might use coping self-statements beneficially: 1. preparing for a stressful experience, 2. dealing with the stressful experience; 3. dealing with the anxiety of being overwhelmed in the midst of the stressful experience; and 4. rewarding yourself after it's all over. A few examples of coping self-statements which might be pertinent to each of the four situations follow, but you're encouraged to adapt these statements to your own personality to make the method even more effective.

In preparing for a stressful experience such as firing an employee, the following thoughts might help: "I've successfully done it before: I can do it again. It's the best thing to do for all concerned. It's got to be done, and I'm the one who can do it best."

While actually firing the person, these thoughts might give you support: "Relax—I'm not the one being fired. I'm in control. Easy does it. One step at a time. I'm meeting this challenge. Keep breathing rhythmically."

As you face the person's strong negative response to being fired, you might keep these ideas in mind: "It will be over soon. I must keep calm. I expected he (she) would need to ventilate some of his (her) feelings about being fired. I've had to deal with worse situations."

After accomplishing the task of firing the person, try using statements like the following: "Hey, that wasn't so bad. I really was able to do it well. It wasn't nearly as bad as I expected; in fact, it wasn't bad at all. I was too anxious about the whole thing. I'm really making improvements in the technique every time I have to fire someone."

You are reminded that your perception of reality is the controlling factor in determining your response to a situation. Coping self-statements in effect help determine what your perception of a stressful experience will be. By silently repeating these statements to yourself, you help keep in check your level of stress, by feeding yourself positive information, instead of focusing on the negative or stressful aspects of the situation. The coping self-statements help guide you in what you are doing and how you feel about your actions. It's important to develop your own coping self-statements, because you alone best know what will have a calming influence upon you. Keep several key coping self-statements in mind so you will have them readily available when needed (see the workbook in the back of the book). In the midst of the stressful situation, you will need to give 20–40 percent of your attention to your coping self-statements in order to maximize their effectiveness. Although at first, the idea of using coping self-statements may strike you as strange, there is evidence suggesting that they can help you reduce stress and improve performance.

Another way of using your head to control stress is a process called systematic desensitization. Whereas coping self-statements help you control the fear and stress that may arise immediately before, during, and after a confrontation, systematic desensitization is more future oriented, taking place far in advance of the actual stressful experience. The basic idea behind desensitization as applied to stress reduction is to teach you to tolerate intense stress by first exposing you to mild stress and then gradually increasing the stress level as fast as you can handle it. The idea is to expose yourself to these various levels of stress by imagining scenes in which the stress is gradually increased while you remain relaxed.

Crucial to the process of desensitization is your ability to construct a "stress hierarchy," consisting of a series of scenes that progressively lead up to your highest point of stress. For example, you decide to go over the head of your boss to the CEO of your company to demand that he fire your boss because of gross incompetence. To say the least, such a situation could be very risky for you, because he just may fire you if you're not convincing enough. In constructing your "stress hierarchy," the actual moment with your CEO when you reveal your bold idea would constitute the moment of highest stress. Let's say that on a stress thermometer (if there were such a gadget) this moment would register 100 degrees. Once you know what the 100 degree situation would be, reconstruct the events leading up to it according to their degrees on the stress thermometer. It might appear as follows:

Least stressful scene	0. Sitting quietly in my office (0°)
	1. Making the appointment with my CEO (10°)
	2. Waking up the morning of my appointment (20°)
	3. Going to work the morning of my appointment (30°)
	4. Planning my exact words (40°)
	5. Walking over to the CEO's office (50°)
	6. Sitting in the CEO's outer office (60°)
	7. Being told I can enter the office (70°)
	8. Walking into the CEO's office (80°)
	9. Small talk with the CEO (90°)
Most stressful scene	10. Telling the CEO my idea (100°)

When you begin systematic desensitization, you should be as relaxed as possible (the next chapter deals with relaxation techniques). Imagine the least stressful scene in your hierarchy for 15 seconds and then relax as you cease your imagining. Relax by imagining yourself in a setting that is very comfortable for you, such as the beach. Then imagine the next scene for 15 seconds as you remain relaxed. Repeat this process all the way up your stress hierarchy, being careful to monitor the tension in your body. If you find that you're getting tense while imagining a certain scene, stop and retreat to that comfortable picture in your mind. You may have to go back and work at staying relaxed while thinking of a less stressful scene. Go further up the hierarchy only when you know you are capable of staying relaxed. The ultimate aim would be to remain calm while imagining the most stressful scene.

At that point the stress will have been counterconditioned and replaced by feelings of relaxation, and you will discover that there is a transfer effect: Desensitizing yourself to a stressful situation carries over and will enable you to remain calmer and under less stress when you really do face the actual experience itself. (Consult the appropriate section of the workbook to create your own "stress hierarchy.")

Vacations

Taking vacations is another way to control stress. Both short and long vacations are needed periodically. If you are very highly involved in your work, a three-week vacation once a year can do wonders. During the first week, you will probably try to forget about your job, which is still very much on your mind. The second week is probably the time you finally relax and psychologically let go of your work. With the arrival of the third week, you are liable to begin to formulate your plans about what you're going to do when you get back to the office. Thus, if you hadn't taken three weeks, you wouldn't have had the one week of pure vacation. You go through this process of disengagement from the job and eventual re-engagement no matter how long your vacation is.

Minivacations, including the now nationally popular three-day weekend, can be quite beneficial. In Chapter 2, I showed that uninterrupted long-term stress creates distress. Vacations, even very short ones, can break up your current stress load and refresh you enough so that you won't suffer from unrelieved stress. Vacations allow you to get away from the stressors and to recoup your inner resources.

A cautionary note is necessary: Be sure that you use your time off in a way that's relaxing and rejuvenating for you. I sometimes wonder about people who get into their campers on the Friday of a three-day weekend, fight the traffic out of town, and rush pell-mell down the road to beat their neighbors to one of the few unreserved spots at the desired campsite, only to fight the traffic on the way home on Sunday or Monday night. This kind of vacation would appear to create far more stress than it would relieve, yet some people find it to be just the break they need, and the stressors involved are much different from the kind these people face at work. Once again, we're back to the principle of deviation and how people can respond differently to the same stressors.

Sometimes your "vacation" may be as short as a few hours or a morning or afternoon off as you vacate that spot in your life which at the moment is putting you under excessive stress. It's amazing how refreshing such a break can be when you really need it.

Sex and love

Maintaining a healthy sex and love life is also important in reducing stress. Poor sex or no sex—either one is bound to create stress. (In Chapter 4, sexual dysfunctions were mentioned as a symptom of excessive stress.) By the same token, a healthy sex life is a natural way to ease stress. Sexual orgasm is by definition a release of tension throughout the body. This physiological release of tension is an extremely natural release valve for the tensions that build up in you as a result of just living in our ever-changing fast-paced world. If you don't have an acceptable outlet for your sexual drives, you're liable to be compounding any stress load you already have.

Love is a powerful force in human life, especially since it's so closely connected to the sexual dimension of our nature. But the human attributes of love, such as tenderness, caring, caressing, sensitivity, and warmth are certainly more important than the physical act of sexual intercourse. As indicated earlier, sexual experience itself becomes better in relationships where the above-mentioned attributes are present, because these human qualities have a soothing, healing effect upon the wounds that distress may have caused. The emotional support found in sharing genuine love with another person can refresh and nourish the human spirit, and the strength that stems from this unconditional regard for the commitment to each other may aid in reducing stress.

Clarifying your values

Clarifying your own values and making sure your life is in harmony with them helps reduce stress. Like most of us, at one point or another, you may fail to stay in touch with what is really important to you. But if your life isn't congruent with your real values, it's as though you are going against the grain. Behavior that is at cross-purposes with your ideals is bound to increase your stress level. You may not be conscious of this impact, but in time it will eventually take its toll.

What's truly important to you? What's the meaning of life? For what, if anything, would you be willing to die? What are your important goals? What does your checkbook indicate is important to you? What would an objective observer of your life's activities think that your values were? Is your behavior consistent with your values?

Questions such as these should help you become more aware of your own personal values. A number of books on values clarification are widely available to help you with this process. Critical to the values clarification process is first becoming aware of your values. The next step is equally critical—bringing the activities of your life in harmony with your real values.

More needs to be said concerning the usefulness of important goals in your life. If you have goals toward which you are working, you will have a purpose to your life which will give meaning to your existence. Montaigne said, "No wind favors him who has no destined port." A ship at sea with full sails set and a nice wind will never get anywhere if it lacks a destination. We must do more than just set our sails if life is to have its richest possible meaning; we must set our sails toward a specific port.

Both modern and ancient history are replete with examples of men and women who were able to overcome tremendous hardships and obstacles because they were headed for something—they had a goal. Physicians can cite case after case in which people pull through severe injuries or diseases simply because they have a reason for living.

Without goals to give purpose and meaning to life, people just don't pull through. Prisoners of war who have the best chances of successfully enduring torture and inhuman conditions and treatment are those who have important goals which give their lives significance beyond that of mere physical survival.

When your values and your life's activities are in harmony, a kind of natural flow and momentum of inner peace and energy come to you. Put another way, an integrated life provides a stable base from which you can manage various stressors. A few years ago young people referred to those who knew what was important to them and who let their life's activities reflect these values as people who "had it together." Picturesque phrases such as these appropriately characterize the flavor of this particular approach to stress reduction. (See "Clarifying Your Values" in the workbook to help you begin this process.) The results, of course, will only be as good as your input. If you honestly seek to understand what your key values are and seek to discover the amount of harmony between them and your life, it could be an invaluable exercise. But if you approach it lightly, it won't even be worth the effort.

Monitoring life's pace

Assessing your own life to see how fast, stressful, and satisfying it is constitutes a final stress-reduction insight. Periodically, you need to sit down (with your spouse if you're married) and examine the pace at which you're living. Is it comfortable for you? Are you well within your elastic limits, or are you getting bent out of shape by trying to do too much? Are you constantly pressing beyond your threshold point? Are you doing the things you want to do, or are you always attempting to please others and not yourself? What about your social calendar during the week and on weekends? Are you accepting and attending social functions you'd really prefer to avoid? Why?

If, as a result of your introspection, you decide you're going pell-mell at a pace you don't like, what specific actions can you take to make your social life more as you would prefer it to be? Perhaps you need to be more assertive in politely declining invitations you don't want to accept. Perhaps you've got to take the initiative and make sure that what you want to do will actually happen. You do have some control over your life's pace if you'll exercise it.

Selye's tips on stress reduction

Because we have such a highly developed nervous system, we are quite vulnerable to psychological insults from others. From a lifetime of research and practical experience, Selye offers several tips (paraphrased here) for dealing with these insults:

1. Don't waste your time trying to befriend those who don't want to be recipients of your love and friendship.

2. Don't be a perfectionist; strive to do something that is within your capabilities.

3. Don't underestimate the genuine pleasure that can come from the simple things of life.

4. Carefully assess each situation to see whether a syntoxic or catatoxic response will serve you best. Only fight for that which is really worth it.

5. Concentrate on the pleasant side of life and on the activities which can improve your lot. As the old German proverb says, "Imitate the sundial's ways; count only the pleasant days."

6. When you do experience a setback or defeat, reestablish your self-confidence by remembering all your past accomplishments.

7. Don't procrastinate in tackling the unpleasant yet necessary tasks you have to do. Get them over with quickly.

8. Realize that people are unequal in many ways at birth. All people should have access to equal opportunities, and their progress should be evaluated on the basis of their performance. Leaders are leaders only as long as they have the respect and loyalty of their followers.

9. Live in such a way as to earn your neighbor's love, and your life will be a happy one. Selye believes that this adapted version of the Golden Rule (love your neighbor as yourself) is more in line with the way humans really are, i.e., egotistical. He's not against the Golden Rule; he just believes that almost no one can love his neighbor as much as he loves himself. So for him the important thing is to work on perfecting yourself so that you will have some usefulness in society.

The person who has earned his neighbor's love will probably never be destitute.[1]

REFERENCES

1. Hans Selye, *Stress Without Distress* (New York: Signet, 1974).
2. William Glasser, *Reality Therapy* (New York: Harper and Row, 1965).
3. Erich Fromm, *The Art of Loving* (New York: Bantam, 1963).
4. Erik H. Erikson, *Childhood and Society* (New York: W. W. Norton and Company, 1950).
5. Lawrence F. Shaffer and Edward J. Shoben, Jr., *The Psychology of Adjustment* (New York: Houghton-Mifflin, 1956).
6. Hans Selye, *The Stress of Life* (New York: McGraw-Hill Book Company, 1976).
7. Karl E. Weick, "The Management of Stress," *MBA Magazine* (October, 1975).
8. W. Timothy Gallwey, *The Inner Game of Tennis* (New York: Random House, 1974).
9. Sharon Anthony Bower and Gordon H. Bower, *Asserting Your Self* (Menlo Park, California: Addison-Wesley, 1976).

CHAPTER 6

Stress-Reduction Techniques

In the last chapter, I dealt with stress-reduction insights that were both syntoxic and catatoxic approaches to managing stress. In this chapter I will show that the spirit of stress-reduction techniques is essentially syntoxic. Exercise, relaxation, and good nutrition are not likely to help us do away with what is causing us stress, but they will help strengthen us so that we can deal with stressors more effectively. In some cases they can also be seen as a temporary flight from the stressor, but never a permanent flight. The temporary flight ultimately enables you to return to the stressful situation with more composure and strength so you can withstand the stressors or perhaps even attack them. But whichever approach you take, you will be better prepared for it through applying some of the techniques discussed in this chapter.

Exercise

Exercise is one of the very finest stress-reduction techniques you can employ. Ironically, according to our definition of stress as the physiological response of the body to any demand, exercise itself places the body under stress. When you are exercising, you are using a stressful activity to combat the ravages of distress. Of course, if you aren't careful, you could overdo it and cause the exercise to become distressful or harmful. Yet, as long as you are not overdoing the strenuous activity, it can be quite beneficial.

The virtues of exercise are many, and they have been properly extolled by various researchers and authors. The benefits of exercise in combating excessive stress are primarily twofold: 1. Vigorous activity in the proper proportions develops cardiovascular fitness; and 2. exercise forces you to relax when it's all over.

Because cardiovascular disease is the number one killer in this country, the importance of cardiovascular fitness can hardly be overemphasized. Remember that your heart is a muscle and, like any other muscle in the body, it must be used if it is to stay strong and healthy. A heart that is not exercised strenuously on a regular basis will become weak and flabby. The heart is like a high-performance engine in a car: It must be run occasionally at high speeds in order to function best, even under more normal conditions. A well-conditioned heart will help prevent heart disease, and if you should suffer a heart attack anyway, a strong heart will make you two to three times more likely to survive. The heart actually works faster, harder, and less efficiently when you "take it easy" than when you make more demands upon it. Unlike other machines, whose life spans are shortened by increased use, the human body extends its own life the more it's properly used.

Many people think that physical exercise may be good for the young, but that an older person who has lived a sedentary life for so long can't really get into any kind of decent physical condition—it might be harmful. These sentiments are very common, but they are definitely wrong. The human body has a marvelous capacity for adaptation. With few exceptions, if you've adjusted so well to an easy, sedentary life, you can also adjust to an active one. The old saying—"If you don't use it, you'll lose it"—is true. For example, when you have been sick in bed for a week or more, your muscles adapt to not being used, so that when you finally get out of bed you are very weak, although you will regain your natural strength in a short time. The adjustment capability of the body works both ways.

At this point several warnings must be sounded regarding the pursuit of cardiovascular fitness through vigorous activity. If you are over 35 years old or have been inactive for some time, you should get the approval of your physician before resuming or undertaking a physical fitness program for the first time. Many physicians will insist upon a stress test—taking an electrocardiogram while stressing the heart by having the patient run on a treadmill. Stress tests are designed in part to detect clogged arteries that could lead to heart attacks, yet the test itself isn't totally reliable because it's possible that a small artery might not be picked up accurately. Besides, some people may place too much confidence in their good EKGs and thus throw caution to the wind in an effort to get in shape overnight. Nothing could be more dangerous, because they could precipitate the very thing they are trying to avoid—a heart attack.

It is well known that a weak heart may be very vulnerable to acute short-term stress, be it emotionally or physically caused. If you should go out and run vigorously for the first time in years, you could shock your heart while it is in a weakened condition by forcing it to pump blood at what might be called an overload rate. If this overload rate were to continue long enough or go high enough, your heart might not be able to take such distress, and it would give up. Many experts believe that it's actually more dangerous to exercise vigorously only once a week than it is not to exercise at all, because the shock may be too much for a heart that is out of shape. If with similar heart conditions you should experience emotional distress, the same phenomenon could occur.

Dr. Kenneth H. Cooper has described a typical case where emotionally induced stress precipitated a fatal heart attack. While working in a hospital he was summoned to treat a patient who was having a heart attack. Although an attempt was made to screen out the noise created during this procedure, the frantic activity was obvious to the other patients on the ward. After successfully completing his treatment of the heart-attack patient, Dr. Cooper saw another patient—an asthmatic—suddenly keel over and die. This patient's heart ceased functioning because of the emotional trauma on the ward. Hormones caused her heart to work too fast for too long a period. Absolutely nothing had been wrong with her heart except that it had been out of condition.

The benefits of achieving cardiovascular fitness—through running, for example—are well known: In sufficient quantities, running improves the efficiency of the lungs, increases the available supply of blood for carrying oxygen to all parts of the body, lowers blood pressure, improves general muscle tone, relaxes the digestive system, extends the vascular system by creating additional blood vessels, and above all strengthens the heart. Improved cardiovascular fitness also correlates with a reduction in levels of glucose, cholesterol, triglycerides, uric acid, body fat, weight, and heart rate.

To be objective, an opposing cautionary point of view from Dr. Meyer Friedman should be noted. Dr. Friedman doesn't dispute the above claims, which essentially indicate that a cardiovascular fitness program started early in life is a good preventive measure against heart disease. His concern is that no one has yet been able to demonstrate conclusively that vigorous activity, such as running, can *undo* damage that may have already occurred to your arteries. Thus, especially middle-aged and older people who may already have partially clogged arteries (which don't always show up on an EKG) may be risking quite a bit by starting to jog. We don't fully understand why plaque, which can be likened to scar tissue, builds up on the inner lining of the artery walls, but it does. With time, cholesterol and other fatty deposits may attach themselves to the plaque on the artery wall, gradually reducing the amount of space through which blood can flow. Apparently, some people are more prone to this build-up than others are. In fact, in some cases infants upon whom autopsies had to be performed were discovered to have plaque-lined arteries. Dr. Kenneth H. Cooper accepts Dr. Friedman's contention that the ability of exercise to open clogged arteries has not yet been confirmed, but Dr. Cooper goes on to say: "But there *is* overwhelming evidence that aerobic exercise will not only work to *prevent* or delay the onset of heart disease, but also help you *survive* a heart attack."[1] The evidence supports the claim that active people are roughly three times as likely to survive a heart attack as are inactive people. Perhaps the importance of exercise is established even more solidly by the dramatic fact that for 40 percent of all heart attack victims, their first symptom of heart disease is the sudden death brought on by the victim's first, last, and only attack.

Let's compare the hearts of two people who are at rest for a 24-hour period. One person has a well-conditioned heart with a resting pulse rate of 60 beats per minute; the other person has a deconditioned heart with a resting pulse rate of 80 beats per minute. The first person's heart will beat 86,400 times in 24 hours, whereas the second person's heart will beat 115,200 times. So even at rest, the difference in the two is almost 30,000 beats per day! That's quite a difference, especially when you realize that with normal activities the deconditioned heart will have to work much harder than the conditioned one. At rest two individuals will pump approximately the same amounts of blood in one minute regardless of age, sex, or physical condition, but the well-conditioned individual will do it easier and with greater efficiency. Conditioned hearts beat more slowly because more blood is being pumped with each stroke. Almost all great distance runners have a pulse rate of 60 beats per minute or lower.

Your pulse is one of the very best indicators of your overall physical condition. Technically, it is nothing more than a wave of blood pushed through your arterial system each time the heart contracts. It's a measure neither of blood pressure nor of the amount of blood leaving the heart; it's simply an indication of how many times your heart is beating against the column of blood already in your circulatory vessels. Wherever a large artery is close to the skin surface, you can feel your pulse. The neck and wrist are two common spots where it can easily be felt. The neck has two carotid arteries. (Don't feel both at the same time because you could diminish the flow of blood to your brain!) Pulse rates vary tremendously. What's normal for you may not be normal for another. You should find out your normal resting pulse rate, because being aware of how soon your heart returns to its normal pulse after vigorous exercise is one of the best safeguards against exercising more strenuously than your condition warrants. For example, if the rate doesn't return to within 10 beats of your resting rate within 15 minutes after ceasing to exercise, you probably should reduce the strenuousness of your activity until your heart becomes stronger.

To check your pulse, put two fingers (not the thumb) on either your wrist or neck. After finding the pulse, count the number of beats for six seconds. By adding a zero to this number you will have the number of beats per minute. The average pulse rates for men are 72-76 beats a minute; for women, the average rates are 75-80. Rates as low as 50 and as high as 100 can still be in the normal range, but in general, the lower the pulse, the healthier the individual. If your resting heart rate is higher than 80, it is likely to be suggestive of poor conditioning. Dr. Laurence E. Morehouse and Leonard Gross report that "the mortality rate for men and women with pulse rates over 92 is four times greater than for those with pulse rates less than 67.[2]

There are many good books on how to develop cardiovascular fitness, and you would do well to consult one for more detailed instructions. When you examine the various approaches, you will find that most theorists agree that three ingredients are essential for any training program to be effective: First, you must find an exercise which is rhythmic enough that you can sustain it for 15 to 20 minutes; second, the exercise must be vigorous enough to sustain your heart rate at between 70 and 85 percent of its capacity for the entire period of time; and third, you must exercise a minimum of three times a week.

Obviously, you should not start out by engaging in some activity that will keep your heart close to its maximal level. It might be better to begin by raising your pulse rate to only 60 percent of capacity, and as you become more fit you could increase it to 70 and finally 85 percent of your maximal attainable heart rate. Going beyond this point won't help you, and it could hurt you. A simple way to estimate your maximal pulse rate is to subtract your age from the number 220. For example, a 40-year-old man would have a top pulse rate of 180. To determine 60 percent of this rate you would simply multiply .60 by 180, which would equal 108. You would start by being sure that your chosen activity got your pulse up to 108 and that you sustained it at that level for at least 15–20 minutes. Of course, as your conditioning improved, you would strive to stay in the 70–85 percent zone. Figure 8 shows the average normal heart rate for each group. There are individual variations in maximal heart rates, so these figures are just averages. In the midst of your exercising you should stop periodically and take your pulse to be sure that it's high enough, yet not too high. As you get into better condition you will find that you have to exert more energy to raise your heart rate to the desired level.

Any activity that involves the body fully and meets the above requirements can be used. Jogging can do it. If you take up jogging, be sure to invest in good shoes, and try to run on grass rather than on hard surfaces, which are much more stressful on the joints. Swimming is particularly good as you grow older, because the buoyancy of the water is quite a bit easier on your joints than is pounding the hard pavement. Because the aging process itself brings about loss of tissue elasticity, the jarring impact of running may give additional stress to

Figure 8. Maximal attainable heart rate and target zone.*

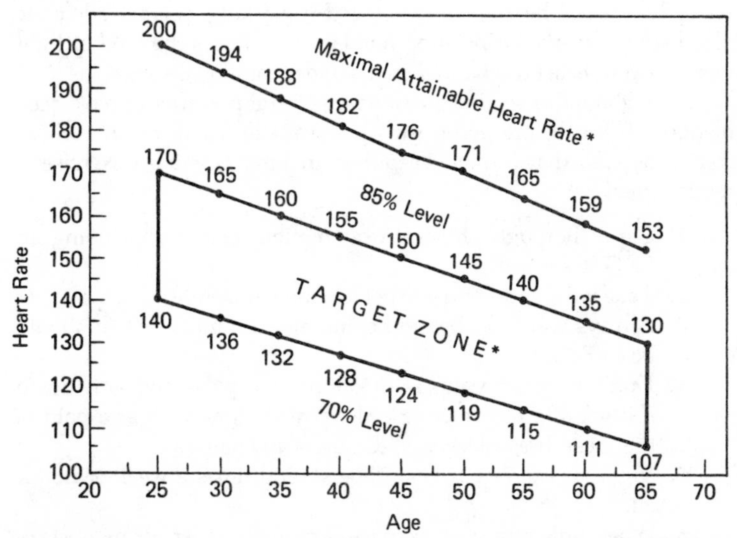

Source: Dr. Lenore R. Zohman, *Beyond Diet: Exercise Your Way to Fitness and Heart Health* (CPC International Inc., 1974), p. 15.

*These numerical values are "average" values for age. It should be noted that one third of the population may differ from these values.

less resilient joints, but this would not be the case with swimming. Ironically, movement, or staying active, is the best way to minimize the debilitating side effects of growing older.

An emotionally induced heart rate (such as one that occurs with sexual arousal), as opposed to one raised through physical activity, does not produce cardiovascular fitness—there just isn't enough muscle involvement. When your heart rate is up due to emotional causes, your muscles aren't pumping a lot of blood back to your heart as they do when you're working out vigorously. To develop the heart needs a lot of blood against which to squeeze. You can feel the difference by first putting a tight fist into the palm of your hand and squeezing it, then putting a weak, limp hand into your palm and squeezing it, too. The difference should be noticeable: The first time you can feel the resistance; the second time, there is very little resistance. This illustrates how your heart gets stronger by working against adequate blood supplies—the weak, limp hand in the palm is the kind of light workout your heart receives when it's under emotional stress.

Throughout this section on exercise, several precautions have been mentioned, but before going further I want to list them, as well as some others, so that you will keep them in mind as you use exercise to reduce stress.

1. Get a thorough physical examination, perhaps including an EKG stress test.
2. Take it easy; don't try to get in shape overnight.
3. Always warm up before beginning—a minute or two should be sufficient.
4. Don't overexert yourself. Monitor your pulse and slow down if it goes up too much. Heed warning signs such as a pain in the chest, breathlessness, dizziness and nausea.
5. Vigorous exercise is best done several times a week or not at all.
6. When finishing your exercise, gradually taper off by observing a five-minute cooling-down period.
7. If your heart rate doesn't return to within 10 beats of your normal resting rate within 15 minutes after you stop exercising completely, reduce the vigor of your activity the next time.
8. Keep plenty of fluids in your body.
9. Don't exercise at all if you are ill.
10. If you jog, wear good shoes; try to jog on grass; and don't jog downhill because it's terribly hard on your knees.
11. After a heavy meal, wait two hours before exercising.

In addition to helping you attain cardiovascular fitness, which is a deterrent to heart disease, a sound exercise program will help you use stress to defeat distress, because vigorous activity ensures that you'll rest afterwards. Prolonged, uninterrupted stress is the kind that becomes distressful, and the rest that follows exercise is a form of forced relaxation, as your body insists upon its recovery time. Were you not working out at all, you might be constantly caught up in a hectic pace and never allow yourself the time for relaxation. At least exercise forces you to slow down occasionally. Vigorous activity also provides a good vehicle for getting rid of your frustrations and pent-up feelings. When you add it all up, it's no wonder that many cardiologists, the people who should know best, are involved in fitness training programs throughout the country. (To help you assess your own level of fitness, see the workbook in the back of the book.)

Relaxation techniques

Relaxation techniques are one of the more promising stress-reduction techniques available today. A relaxed body is physiologically the opposite of a stressed body. Stress causes various physiological indicators of your body's condition—such as blood pressure, respiration rate, heart rate, brain wave activity, and muscle tone—to increase. When you induce the relaxation response, these and other physiological indicators decrease. Here again, Selye's finding on how uninterrupted stress can become distressful is important: Relaxation breaks up the stress load at least temporarily, and even a short break can be valuable.

RELAXATION VS. COFFEE BREAKS

The ubiquitous coffee break is called a "break" because it helps us get away from the pressures (stressors) of work. But what actually happens on the average coffee break? First, you drink coffee (or tea or soft drinks), whose caffeine acts as a stimulant to your system, and produces additional stress in your body. As was pointed out in Chapter 4, ingesting only 250 mg. of caffeine can cause you to exhibit the same symptoms as people who are suffering from clinical anxiety. (The average cup of coffee contains at least 100 mg. of caffeine and maybe as much as 150 mg.) Much the same can be said for tea and soft drinks, although their caffeine content is slightly less than coffee's.

Second, on the typical coffee break many people smoke. Nicotine acts initially on the body as a stimulant; only later does it have a depressant effect. With the first puff, smokers may be psychologically relaxed, but their heart rates are actually climbing. Third, on coffee breaks, many people eat junk food that has a lot of fat and sugar. These foods, which have little nutritional value, are potentially quite harmful, because they contribute to higher levels of cholesterol and fatty deposits in the bloodstream, which can eventually contribute to hardening of the arteries and to coronary artery disease.

Thus, the traditional coffee break usually serves to *increase* stress in the body rather than to reduce it. A recent study at Eltra Corporation's Converse Rubber Company indicated that relaxation breaks instead of coffee breaks tend to improve workers' overall health and help them get greater satisfaction from their jobs.[3] Two experimental groups took 15-minute relaxation breaks twice a day for two months; two control groups did not. At the end of the study, the experimental groups showed a greater drop in blood pressure, headaches, and sleep problems, as well as improvement in their job satisfaction and in their ability to deal with others.

You may want to consider taking relaxation breaks rather than coffee breaks. If you practice some form of meditation, you could do it in your office. Or you could just go outside and take a short, brisk walk. Whatever method you use, doing something relaxing will probably allow you to come back to your hectic day more refreshed and better able to cope with your job for the rest of the day—far better able than you would have been had you not taken the break. Perhaps in the future, farsighted companies will provide quiet, comfortable rooms for relaxation. (Why not? They already provide vending machines for the traditional coffee break.) Taking relaxation breaks makes use of the priniciple of deviation which Selye so strongly encourages because of its therapeutic value.

MEDITATION AS A FORM OF RELAXATION

Meditation isn't simply a matter of thinking about some concept, religious or otherwise; it is an "exercise" in which you seek to gain mastery over the process of attention. The goal of this mastery is an altered state of consciousness in which you drop your normal way of screening, processing, and classifying the stimuli that come your way and instead perceive those stimuli directly.[4] Concentration is quite important in this process. When you meditate successfully, it's almost as though there has been a temporary shutdown of the information-processing mechanisms of the brain, which are responsible for so much of your stress (remember the importance of your *response* in determining the stressfulness of any stressor).[5] The physiological response that underlies this transcendental awareness is called by some the relaxation response. Eliciting the relaxation response causes the body to counteract the biochemical changes that accompany the fight-or-flight response (see Chapter 2). The obvious benefit of this mechanism is that you can induce the relaxation response (once you learn it) whenever you are confronted with a particularly stressful situation.

There are other benefits as well. Numerous studies show rather clearly that the relaxation response causes the following physiological changes to occur: Oxygen consumption decreases; respiratory rate decreases; heart rate decreases; alpha brain waves (which signify a more relaxed state) increase; blood pressure decreases; and muscle tension decreases.[6] Of course, all these changes are associated with *de*stressing or *un*stressing the body. It is also quite clear that simply sitting quietly with your eyes closed does not elicit the relaxation response. These changes are also different from those that accompany sleep.[7]

Before looking at a number of different approaches that can elicit the relaxation response, we need to make several clarifications.[4] First, meditation is not a panacea that by itself will automatically bring you all you ever wanted out of life, including a reduction in stress. The sources of stress are many and varied. Meditation can help prevent your overreaction to stress, but it's only one part of your total behavior; it can't do everything. Second, as with most activities, your attitude toward meditation will determine whether it works for you. Those who believe that it will work and therefore have positive attitudes toward it are more likely to practice regularly and to experience the benefits. Third, to be effective in eliciting the relaxation response through meditation, you do not need to follow any one "correct" method or adhere to a particular group's religious views. No single technique is known to work best for everybody, and you will probably be attracted to one more than the others. If this proves to be the case, concentrate on that one technique until you can regularly use it to bring about the desired state of physical relaxation.

TRANSCENDENTAL MEDITATION ("TM")

Transcendental Meditation, better known as "TM," was introduced to the United States in 1959 by the Indian teacher, Maharishi Mahesh Yogi. It is by far the best known and most often practiced of the various approaches to meditation. Maharishi chose to use the term transcendental (meaning "going beyond") to signify that TM takes you beyond wakeful experience to a state of restfulness which is also characterized by a heightened sense of alertness.

The technique for practicing TM is surprisingly simple. It involves the repetition of a mantra (a monosyllabic word or sound) for 20 minutes a day twice a day, morning and evening. The mantra, which is especially chosen for you, is supposed to be kept a secret and to help absorb your attention in order to quiet and still the conscious mind. With practice you will be able to achieve a state of heightened awareness in which you are wide awake inside while relatively oblivious to outside stimuli. If in the process of repeating your mantra, other thoughts should come into your mind, you are supposed to let your mind flow over these thoughts and return to your mantra. If you try too hard to prevent such occurrences, you will probably interrupt the process; you have to just "let it happen." The practitioners of TM insist that meditation is natural—it will come if you orient the mind in the right direction and "let it happen."

Practicing TM usually brings the important benefits we mentioned earlier in this chapter. Dr. Herbert Benson of the Harvard Medical School, along with others, has thoroughly documented these results. However, they have also established that other approaches to meditation can also help de-stress the body. (TM has always had an exclusivity and arrogance that bothered some people, and there are other equally valuable approaches to meditation.)

BENSON'S RELAXATION RESPONSE

Herbert Benson's technique for eliciting the relaxation response, which is the underlying physiological condition of all forms of meditation, is built upon four basic components. First, you need a quiet, calm environment that offers the fewest possible distractions. Second, you need some mental device upon which to concentrate so as to keep your attention from outside thoughts, worries, and concerns. While repeating this word or phrase, it helps to pay attention to your normal rhythm of breathing. Third, develop a passive attitude. When distracting thoughts enter your mind, don't worry about them, just disregard them and redirect your attention to your mental device. Fourth, place yourself in a comfortable position, one that doesn't create any unnecessary muscular tension. Lying down is usually not best because it's easier to fall asleep that way than if you are sitting. Just be comfortable and relaxed.

The following technique for eliciting the relaxation response is the same one used by Benson at Harvard's Thorndike Memorial Laboratory. It has been found to produce the same physiological changes that TM does. The technique is as follows[6]:

1. Sit quietly in a comfortable position.
2. Close your eyes.
3. Deeply relax all your muscles, beginning at your feet and progressing up to your face. Keep them relaxed.
4. Breathe through your nose. Become aware of your breathing. As you breathe out, say the word, "one," silently to yourself. For example, breathe in . . . out, "one"; in . . . out, "one;" and so on. Breathe easily and naturally.
5. Continue for 10 to 20 minutes. You may open your eyes to check the time, but do not use an alarm. When you finish, sit quietly for several minutes, at first with your eyes closed and later with your eyes open. Do not stand up for a few minutes.
6. Do not worry about whether you are successful in achieving a deep level of relaxation. Maintain a passive attitude and permit relaxation to occur at its own pace. When distracting thoughts occur, try to ignore them by not dwelling upon them, and return to repeating "one." With practice, the response should come with little effort. Practice the technique once or twice daily, but not within two hours after any meal, since the digestive processes seem to interfere with the elicitation of the Relaxation Response.

Every person has the capacity to elicit the relaxation response whether through the above simple method of Benson's or by some other approach. The response itself is an innate one. According to Benson, the voluntary, regular elicitation of this response "can counterbalance and alleviate the effects of the environmentally induced, but often inappropriate, fight-or-flight response."[8]

YOGA

Yoga has been one of the most successful methods of decreasing stress through a mixture of mental and physical approaches. Actually there are many forms of yoga, but in the West, hatha yoga is probably the best known and the most popular. Yoga literally means union or fusing. It aims to unite mind and body to bring inner tranquility. The name hatha is derived from Sanskrit (as is yoga) and combines ha, the female principle, and tha, the male principle. Hatha yoga is "unisex" yoga and enables both men and women to gain control of mind and body. Practitioners of yoga claim that it brings not only mental calm and relief from stress, but also better health, more vigor, and a clearer, more alert mind.

In his research Dr. Chandra Patel has discovered that patients who practice yoga can reduce their blood pressure, along with their need for drug therapy.[4] His findings actually show that these reductions lasted between sessions and, in fact, as long as the patients continued to practice yoga. Yoga involves various body postures (asanas) and breathing exercises. The particular posture used by Dr. Patel's patients was the posture of shavasana, better known as the corpse pose. Anyone can practice it; it doesn't require the progression through training that would be required to achieve the lotus position. Although the following description may sound simple, don't be deceived—it does require some practice.

To adopt the corpse pose, begin by lying on your back with your feet comfortably apart and pointed outward. Allow your arms to lie alongside your body at a comfortable distance from the body with your palms up and your eyes closed. Focus on various regions of the body, beginning with your feet and moving upwards, and relax these regions progressively. Imagine that you are sinking into the carpet. Breathe naturally, using the diaphragm only. When you are using diaphragmatic breathing (called the "breath of life" or "pranayama"), your abdominal wall will rise and fall with each breath and your chest wall will remain still. When you are quite relaxed as a result of relaxing your muscles and breathing properly, then you can meditate by mentally repeating a sound or word such as "om" or "one." This repetition will help to keep worries from entering your mind. The time required for this activity is 15–20 minutes at least once a day.

As with other meditative approaches it is best not to eat before engaging in yoga. You should also find a quiet, comfortable spot, perhaps with a thickly carpeted floor. Don't breathe too deeply and rapidly—you might induce a light-headed feeling due to hyperventilation. You should avoid going to sleep; bringing your feet closer together will help fight off any drowsiness. For the corpse posture described above, it was suggested that you close your eyes, although meditative traditions differ on the issue of opening or closing the eyes. Zen Buddhists, for example, keep the eyes partially open because they believe that closed eyes bring on drowsiness and symbolize a withdrawal from life. By cultivating an attentive but unfocused gaze, they try to maintain alertness along with a low-frequency brain-wave pattern.

Contrary to popular opinion, yoga is not designed to be a painful set of body contortions. It is true that in hatha yoga there are a number of positions through which you may progress, beginning with the simplest and moving to the more complex. But the idea is *not* to cause yourself great pain; in fact, if a particular position is painful, you should stop. The purpose of the various positions is to increase the mobility and suppleness of your body, but only gradually. Most people who think it's painful probably started off by trying to get into the lotus position. The yoga exercises also attempt to benefit particular regions of the body by relaxing them, which in turn helps calm the mind. So, through deep and rhythmic breathing, body positioning, and mental focusing, yoga brings about a harmony and oneness between mind and body that tends to bring inner harmony and serenity to the spirit. And for the small amount of time it requires, that's quite a payoff.

AUTOGENIC TRAINING

Autogenic training is a deep-relaxation technique which was developed by Johannes H. Schultz, a German psychiatrist. Through a combination of specific exercises and autohypnosis, autogenic training brings about deep mental and physical states of relaxation. On the basis of his own previous work with subjects who entered hypnotic states of consciousness, Schultz knew that these subjects experienced two powerful physical sensations: a generalized feeling of warmth throughout the entire body, and a feeling of heaviness in the torso and limbs. The warm feeling is the psychological perception of the dilation of the arteries, which occurs with relaxed states; the feeling of heaviness results from the actual relaxation of the muscles. Schultz's concept of autogenic training was meant to design exercises so that people could teach themselves to bring about these two sensations and thus achieve the state of "passive concentration" comparable to the goal of other methods of meditation. Schultz had seen how his patients who underwent hypnosis experienced lessened fatigue, tension, and psychosomatic disorders, and he wanted to enable others to experience the same benefits without having to go into hypnosis therapy.

Autogenic training begins with exercises designed to bring about physical relaxation. As with most other meditative approaches, you should first get into a comfortable setting with a minimum of distractions. Three positions are available: lying down (almost identical to the corpse position in yoga), sitting in a reclining chair, and sitting comfortably in a straight-backed chair. The first thing you should do is to relax. Imagine that there is a string attached to the top of your head, that it goes to the ceiling, and that you are being pulled into an upright position. Now imagine that the string is cut and you collapse and become as limp as a rag doll (although don't collapse too much—it may interfere with your breathing). Once in this loose and limp state, you will be ready to begin the physical exercises.

First, you should *passively* give your attention to your dominant arm. (Don't work at it too hard; just let it happen.) While becoming aware of this arm, you should silently repeat the phrase, "My right arm is heavy," three to six times for 30–60 seconds. After this time, stir around vigorously and open your eyes, then flex your arms and move different parts of your body. This movement is called a cancellation activity. Your right arm will probably retain some residual feeling of heaviness. Repeat the above procedure four times, allowing a minute between each repetition.

The next step is to duplicate this exercise with your other arm. After getting your other arm to feel heavy, begin to say, "Both arms are heavy," and go through the sequence once more. Be sure to cancel or stir around and flex the different parts of your body after each exercise. An effective cancellation phrase might be, "Arms firm, breathe deeply, open eyes." As you work on your arms, you will most likely begin to feel heaviness in other parts of the body as well. This feeling is desirable and important. After working on your arms, you should go through the same procedures with your legs, beginning with your dominant leg.

The second stage of the physical part of autogenic training involves inducing feelings of warmth. Some warm feelings probably already have been generated, but to produce even more, go through the same progression as you did for the induction of heavy feelings. Remember to use the cancellation technique between each series of instructions to yourself.

The third stage is cardiac regulation. Here again the procedure is very similar, although there are slight variations in this case. The formula to repeat is "heartbeat calm and regular." Repeat this phrase for a longer time (90–180 seconds) with your hand over your heart. Do it four times and be sure to use a cancellation phrase such as "eyes open, breathe deeply" between the exercises. The fourth stage focuses on respiration. The procedure here is the same as for the cardiac regulation, except that you repeat to yourself, "It breathes me."

The fifth stage is intended to bring about warm sensations in the abdominal region. The surface of the skin is not what you're trying to warm up; you are trying to imagine a warmth deep in your lower abdominal cavity, or in your solar plexus. Some find it helpful to put their hands there and to imagine a sensation of heat radiating outward from that area. The words to use are, "My solar plexus is warm." Repeat the words during four different periods, using your cancellation technique between each period. This particular exercise should help calm down the central-nervous-system activity.

The sixth and final stage of the physical part of autogenic training entails using the phrase, "My forehead is cool." A lying-down posture is recommended, since dizziness may be experienced. Begin slowly by repeating the phrase for 10–20 seconds and eventually work up to four repetitions of 30–60 seconds each.

After a few months of practice, you can learn to advance through these six stages in a matter of a few minutes. Then you will be ready for what comes after the physical exercises—autogenic meditation. This advanced phase of autogenic training involves picturing and holding certain images in the mind. It is believed that you can achieve focused awareness through visualization while remaining aloof from ordinary thoughts and emotions. You begin this meditative phase of autogenic training by rolling your eyeballs upward and inward as though you were looking at the center of your forehead. Once in this position, you go through a series of visions which you bring to your mind. For more information on these visualization exercises, see Kenneth R. Pelletier's *Mind as Healer, Mind as Slayer,* from which I have drawn much of this material.

SELF-HYPNOSIS AND AUTOSUGGESTION

A sense of the mysterious has always surrounded hypnotism, largely because of misunderstandings caused by the theatrical tricks of stage hypnotists, so before I go any further, it is necessary to dispel several misconceptions about hypnosis.[5] First, hypnosis is not the same as sleep. Instead of being unconscious and unaware in a hypnotic state, you actually have tremendous awareness and sensitivity. Second, you don't lose control of yourself under hypnosis; what you do lose is the conscious *feeling* of control, yet you are still in control to handle any emergencies that may arise. Third, you don't enter a hypnotic state because a spell was cast upon you by a skilled hypnotist—you allow *yourself* to slip into the state; it's an ability you already have to some extent.

Hypnosis is "the altered state of consciousness that results from focusing awareness on a set of suggestions and allowing oneself to be receptive to those suggestions—all while allowing free reign to one's powers of imagination."[5] There are various levels of hypnotic states, but we are concerned only with alteration of consciousness that facilitates relaxation and autosuggestions (suggestions made by you to yourself). The goal of relaxation is worthy in and of itself, as we have seen repeatedly. Autosuggestions can help you change your thinking and behavior in ways that will lessen your stress, because under hypnosis you are more receptive to having your mental computer reprogrammed in useful directions.

Two methods are typically used in self-hypnosis: the eye-fixation method and the eye-roll technique. To use the eye-fixation method, get comfortable and focus your attention on some stationary object. As you concentrate on it, silently tell yourself that your eyelids are getting heavier and heavier and that pretty soon they will close and you'll be very relaxed, yet fully aware. Repeat this suggestion every 60 seconds. When the eyelids are ready, let them close. Slowly take a deep breath, hold it for 10 to 15 seconds, then exhale. As you breathe comfortably, say the word "relax" when you exhale each time.

In using the eye-roll method, roll your eyes inward and upward and look at the center of the top of your forehead. While holding this position, close your eyes and take a deep breath; hold it; release it; and let your eyes return to their normal position. Imagine that your body is becoming heavier and heavier, warmer and warmer. Take each of the major sets of muscles in your body and in turn imagine these sensations of heaviness and warmth. This process will bring on greater relaxation. Now you are ready to deepen your light trance.

Take another deep breath, hold it, and as you begin to exhale, say the word "deeper." Imagine that you are on a slow-moving escalator going down as you say, "I am going still deeper and deeper." Remember that you are in control at all times. At any moment you can come out of this light trance by saying, "I'm coming out," and then opening your eyes. Some prefer to come out more gradually by saying, "When I get to the count of five, my eyes will open."

Normally, at this point you would be very relaxed. If not, you may suggest to yourself that you are relaxing more with each exhalation. Now is the time to give yourself self-change suggestions. Here are six guidelines that may help you formulate good suggestions:

1. The more you repeat the suggestion, the more effective it will be.

2. Be positive rather than negative. Say to yourself, "I am going to be more relaxed as I face deadlines in the future," rather than "I shouldn't get so tense over meeting deadlines."

3. Don't expect drastic changes overnight. Anticipate progress in degrees.

4. See yourself gradually feeling better about yourself, rather than saying that you are going to *try* to feel better about yourself. The latter approach implies that your chances of changing are not very good.

5. Avoid phrasing your suggestions as orders. Instead of saying, "I must," say "I choose to." Resistance to taking orders from anyone, including oneself, seems built into most of us.

6. Try to develop a visual image that reinforces your suggestion. Imagine yourself being relaxed as you face an important deadline. Imagery can be very powerful. There's little doubt that you can reduce stress through self-hypnosis and autosuggestion if you are open and receptive to the idea. However, if you have a skeptical or negative

attitude toward hypnosis or toward any of the different kinds of meditation discussed to this point, then progressive muscular relaxation may be tailor-made for you.

PROGRESSIVE MUSCLE RELAXATION

Progressive muscle relaxation, first discovered by Edmund Jacobson, is a method for inducing relaxation initially in the body—and eventually in the mind—by employing a series of sequential physical exercises.[9] In these exercises, one muscle group in the body (for example, the hand and forearm) is contracted or held tense for about seven seconds and then completely and abruptly relaxed for 20 to 60 seconds. This tension-release pattern is repeated again and then sequentially repeated with various muscle groups throughout the entire body.

Jacobson believed that tense muscles and emotions go hand in hand. By learning to relax muscles through specific exercises, you can find mental relaxation as well. Jacobson's thinking was right in line with modern thinking about psychosomatic diseases: The mind and the body are integrally related; a change in either's condition will affect the other as well. It may strike you as strange that by first tensing a muscle and then releasing it, you can induce a more relaxed state in that muscle, but it's true—and what's more, it has been shown that this form of relaxation can reduce stress.

One of the by-products of training in progressive muscle relaxation is that you can learn to become more sensitive to rising tension levels in your body before the tension gets so great that it causes pain. The more aware you are of how relaxed muscles feel, the more sensitivity you'll have toward them as they start to become tense. As the tension mounts and you become aware of it, you can do something about it before it gets out of control. The following instructions on progressive muscle relaxation include some deep breathing and mental imagery techniques as well, neither of which was originally emphasized by Jacobson.

When instructed to take a deep breath, be sure to involve your diaphragm. Most people take a deep breath by raising their upper chest, but you can take a deeper breath by pushing down and out on the diaphragm, which is the muscle along the bottom of your rib cage. If you start by filling the lower chest cavity, you can expand to the upper area of the lungs; but if you fill the top part of the lungs first, you won't be able to take in more air below. Good singers and speakers have long known this secret.

Rhythmic breathing will also help you keep yourself calmer in stressful situations. It doesn't matter whether your respirations are 5 a minute or 20: The simultaneous, rhythmic working of the upper and lower chest in exhaling and inhaling keeps the body more relaxed than it would otherwise be when faced with stress. It is generally recommended that you practice progressive muscle relaxation at least once a day. It can be done lying down or sitting comfortably. The instructions given here assume that you are sitting down. I believe that you can profitably engage in this activity even when driving home in your car, but with one exception—you shouldn't close your eyes! Some people practice it at work as part of their relaxation break. Some tape the instructions (or have someone with a calm voice tape them) and then listen to the tape. Nothing is sacrosanct about these particular instructions—once you get the idea, you can make up your own.

First, sit down with your eyes closed, make yourself as comfortable as you can, and try to relax to the best of your ability. Push competing thoughts out of your mind and just let go. Remember, the body is naturally inclined to relax if you will just get out of the way and let it happen. Don't work at relaxing; it will come as you let go. Think of some nice, comfortable, relaxing scene. Throughout this exercise keep the scene in the back of your mind. The particular scene is unimportant; just pick one that speaks of tranquility to you. It might be a picture of you on the beach on a warm, sunny day, lying on the sand basking in the warm rays of the sun, sinking deeper and deeper into the sand as you feel warm and relaxed all over. Or perhaps for you, the relaxing scene is in the mountains as you lie on the bank of a lake or of a mountain stream, gazing through a grove of pine trees into the blue sky.

While you are imagining yourself in this peaceful, elysian scene, take a deep breath and hold it (each deep breath in these instructions should be about seven seconds), then slowly exhale. Each time you exhale, imagine the tension leaving your body. Now once again take a deep breath, hold it, and slowly exhale. As you exhale, you can begin to feel your whole body relaxing.

Now direct your attention to the muscles of your right hand and forearm. With your arm flat on the arm of your chair or in your lap, clench your right fist and keep it clenched for about seven seconds. (This length of time will be the same throughout the exercise whenever any muscles are tensed.) Become aware of the tension in the forearm. Now relax completely. Each time you are instructed to relax a muscle, do it immediately—not gradually. Notice the difference between the tensed state and the relaxed state. Enjoy the relaxed state (each time allow 20 to 60 seconds for this enjoyment of the relaxed state). Now, once again, tense your right hand and forearm by clenching your right fist. Focus on the tension, hold it, then abruptly let go and relax.

Now flex your right bicep muscle, but be sure to keep your wrist limp. As you tense this muscle and hold it, you can feel it becoming hotter. Now let your arm relax and flop down like a limp washcloth. Notice the contrast between the muscles when they're tense and when they're relaxed. Repeat this tension-release cycle for your upper right arm. Upon completing the cycle, go through the same sequence with your left hand and left bicep muscle. Be sure to do two tension-release cycles for each muscle group. At the conclusion of these steps, remind yourself, if you've forgotten, of the pleasant environment you're picturing yourself in, then take another deep breath, and exhale.

At this point direct your attention to your forehead. Wrinkle your forehead and make the lines appear by raising your eyebrows. Keep them tensed, tighter and tighter. Now relax, and imagine the lines smoothing out and disappearing. Repeat these steps, then take a nice deep breath, hold it, and exhale. Frown and crease your brow, tighter and tighter. Hold it, and relax. Repeat this entire tension-release procedure for your eye muscles, your jaw, your lips, your neck muscles, your shoulders, your stomach muscles, your buttocks, your thighs, and your calves, until you've gone through the major muscle groups in your body.

When you have finished the entire process, once again imagine that you are in that comfortable environment, feeling very relaxed all over. Now take an extra deep breath, hold it, and slowly exhale. You should now be able to enjoy complete relaxation and tranquility. Enjoy this state for a while and when you are ready to conclude the exercise, arouse yourself gradually. Gently move a limb or two and stir about as you open your eyes.

BIOFEEDBACK

You will recall that stress tends to raise blood pressure, brain wave activity, and heart rate, and to increase muscle tension and skin sweating. Although for years it was thought that you couldn't control these automatic functions of the autonomic nervous system, we now know differently: You can control them with your mind. Biofeedback is a way of helping you control one or more of these processes. A biofeedback machine simply gives you feedback on how much stress there is in a certain part of your body. The machine itself doesn't change the temperature in your fingers, for example; it just monitors the temperature and feeds this information back to you. You create whatever change there is. The more relaxed or de-stressed your fingers are, the warmer they will be. It's natural for the body to want to relax; biofeedback machines just measure *how* relaxed certain parts of our body are.

Muscle tension is measured by an electromyograph (EMG). The EMG records the degree of tension in whatever muscle group the electrode pads are measuring. This information is fed back to you in the form of a tone. The louder the tone, the greater the tension; the lower the tone, the less the tension. Other well-known biofeedback devices consist of those used to measure brain wave activity (electroencephalograph or EEG machine), those used to measure the electrical conductivity of the skin (galvanic skin response or GSR), and those used to measure skin temperature (a mood ring is a crude temperature-oriented biofeedback device). Feedback is given in various ways—an audible tone, a light signal, or a deviation on a meter dial.

When biofeedback first became popular, it was heralded by some as "instant electronic yoga," because low brain-wave activity is characteristic of meditators and because you can learn to lower brain-wave activity through biofeedback training, thus bringing about deep relaxation through biofeedback regulation of EEG frequencies. The problem with this reasoning is that a biofeedback machine will help you to control only the specific function it is monitoring. Deep relaxation is not just low brain wave activity; it is an integrated combination of a number of bodily processes. Studies have shown, however, that high levels of stress can be fought effectively with a combination of techniques designed to induce deep relaxation (for example, yoga) and the specific control of a particular area in which stress is manifest, such as high blood pressure.[4] Of course, biofeedback works well on specific disorders such as hypertension. We don't understand how people lower their blood pressure through biofeedback, but we do know that it can be done.

One potential problem with using biofeedback machines—other than that they are expensive or cumbersome—is that you may use one of these devices before finding out exactly what is really bothering you. For example, suppose that you are plagued by persistent headaches and you buy an EMG machine to help you get rid of the headaches. You are assuming that you have a muscle-tension headache—but what if you really have a brain tumor? Be sure you know what your symptoms mean before setting out to correct them. Obviously, the best advice is always to consult your doctor first. In fact, to achieve maximal results, it would be best to work with your physician and with a specialist in the kind of relaxation training you desire. With the exception of progressive muscle-relaxation training, all the other kinds of techniques mentioned here will probably be far more effective if you get more thorough instruction.

Good nutrition

Although the exact relationship between nutrition and stress is unknown, the American people are more conscious of good nutrition now than perhaps they have ever been, and probably with good reason. Nutritionally unsound habits can cause disease. Excessive intake of fat, sugar, salt, cholesterol, and caffeine are widely recognized as contributing to poor health and to certain diseases, particularly hardening of the arteries, diabetes, hypertension, and heart disease.

It is reasonable to believe that in a limited way we are the product of our digestion. We are, in part, what we eat, because it's only through eating and drinking that we sustain our bodies. I strongly suspect that we are going to find that a body that has been made healthy and strong by proper intake of essential nutrients is a body that will not suffer from certain nutritionally related diseases, and will be better able to survive stress, just as a well-conditioned heart is more likely to survive a heart attack.

Although the American public is more nutritionally aware today than before, the average American is still by and large a nutritional illiterate. Recently, I asked a group of professional people to name the four basic food groups and how many adult servings they were to have each day from each group. I was amazed to find that not one individual of the 25 people there could name all four of the groups, much less the proper daily portions. Just in case you've forgotten, the four basic food groups are as follows (the number of recommended adult servings per day is shown in parentheses): the milk group (2), the meat group (2), the fruit and vegetable group (4), and the bread and cereal group (4).

It's unfortunate that most Americans know as little as they do about good nutrition. Most of us were brought up to be junk food junkies: We are addicted to foods that are high in fat, in refined sugar content, and in calories, but very deficient in the most important area —nutrients. (It is ironic that as most civilizations have "advanced," their diets have deteriorated!) Forty percent of the average American's calories are obtained from fat.[10] There is great controversy over whether unsaturated fats are better for you than are saturated fats, yet the evidence strongly suggests that most of us would be far better off with a lot fewer fats—regardless of the type—than we now ingest.

The average American shows a level of cholesterol of about 200 mg. for each 100 cu. cm. of blood. Harvard nutritionist Frederick J. Stare says that cholesterol levels start to get dangerous at about 230 mg. Thus, the average American is already flirting with danger. Cholesterol is a blood lipid, or fat, that is synthesized in the liver. It is essential for many bodily functions, particularly those of your brain. Excessive blood cholesterol possibly contributes to hardening of the arteries and almost certainly aggravates an already existing condition. Cholesterol is a fat, or lipid, found in different kinds of fat–protein combinations in our blood. For instance, high-density lipoproteins seem to protect blood vessels, whereas low-density lipoproteins tend to accelerate development of plaque. Interestingly enough, high-density lipoproteins appear to be enhanced by exercise. Some evidence suggests that low-fat diets are far more effective in fighting atherosclerosis than are low-cholesterol diets alone. Cholesterol is contained in many of our favorite animal food products, but is only one form of dietary fat.

The average American consumes more than 126 pounds of sugar a year. This statistic surprises many people, because they are often unaware of how much sugar is put into most processed foods. Excessive sugar in the body can lead to a number of problems, such as obesity, tooth decay, diabetes, high levels of blood fat, and atherosclerosis. The body, however, does need sugar, although it benefits most when it gets its fuel from complex carbohydrates rather than from refined sugar or simple carbohydrates.

Simple sugars, such as honey, increases a blood fat called triglycerides; complex carbohydrates, such as bread, do not have that effect on triglycerides. Like blood cholesterol, blood triglycerides are a risk factor associated with heart disease. Lowering your sprinkled or poured-on sugar intake can reduce your chances of getting heart disease.

It is well known that Americans consume too much salt and that salt can contribute to the development of hypertension. The effects of caffeine have been dealt with earlier, but one additional point should be made—caffeine increases the amount of free fatty acids in the blood.

The question may arise: What about vitamin supplements? Despite claims to the contrary, most nutritionists who stay abreast of the research-based scientific studies do not believe that vitamin supplements are necessary if you eat a well-rounded diet. The "megavitamin craze" is even potentially dangerous because massive doses of such vitamins as A and D can become toxic to your system because they are fat-soluble and can be stored in your body for long periods. Massive doses of vitamin C may slightly decrease the frequency and duration of some cold symptoms, but no one has proved that it can keep you from getting the cold in the first place.

In conclusion, when you try to evaluate all the known and unknown aspects of nutrition, it would seem that the wisest course of action would be to lower your intake of fat, sugar, salt, calories, and caffeine; to try to eat the recommended portions from the four basic food groups; and to exercise moderation in all things. Certainly such an approach isn't going to hurt you, and there is a lot of evidence suggesting that it will improve your health considerably.

REFERENCES

1. "Formulas for Fitness: How Aerobics Can Help Your Heart—and the Way You Feel," *Reader's Digest,* January, 1978.
2. *Total Fitness in 30 Minutes a Week* (New York : Pocket Books, 1976), p. 151.
3. *The Wall Street Journal,* December 1, 1977; see also Ruanne K. Peters and Herbert Benson, "Time Out From Tension," *Harvard Business Review,* January–February, 1978.
4. Kenneth R. Pelletier, *Mind as Healer, Mind as Slayer* (New York : Delta, 1977).
5. Robert L. Woolfolk and Frank C. Richardson, *Stress, Sanity and Survival* (New York: Monarch, 1978).
6. Herbert Benson, *The Relaxation Response* (New York: William Morrow and Company Inc., 1975).
7. Herbert Benson, Jamie B. Kotch, Karen D. Crassweller, and Martha M. Greenwood, "Historical and Clinical Considerations of the Relaxation Response," *American Scientist,* July-August 1977.
8. Herbert Benson, "Your Innate Asset for Combating Stress," *Harvard Business Review,* July-August 1974.
9. Edmund Jacobson, *Progressive Relaxation* (Chicago: University of Chicago Press, 1938).
10. Corinne H. Robinson, *Fundamentals of Normal Nutrition* (New York: The Macmillan Company, 1973).

CHAPTER 7

A Final Word About Stress

I frequently get the following questions from people who are obviously suffering from excessive stress: "Can people really change their behavior? Can a Type A person become a Type B? Can a junk food junkie start eating nutritionally sound food and give up sweets and fatty foods? Can an inactive person become active?" My answer always is, "Yes, you can change if you really want to change." The evidence is there if you are willing to look at it. For example, there are many cases in which people with Type A personalities suffer from heart attacks, and upon recovering drastically change their lives. Many of these people have nothing special going for them; if you become aware of how distressed your body is, and if you recognize the harmful potential in such distress, you can become motivated to change, too.

Clearly, I am not suggesting that it is easy to change old habits—but it is possible. One of the more useful ways to assist yourself in bringing about the desired changes in your own life that will help you manage stress better is to use the principles of behavior modification upon yourself. Choose a specific behavior that you want to change, note what your current behavior is and decide on your goal. As you move toward your goal, reward yourself by indulging in some pleasure that you normally don't allow yourself. If you backslide, punish yourself by withholding the reward. For example, let's assume you are overweight by about 20 pounds. You know that being overweight isn't good for you, so you resolve to lose four pounds a month for five months. To lose this amount of weight, you would have to cut your calorie intake by only 250 calories a day and increase your activity level enough to burn up 250 more calories a day than you normally do. Taking into consideration that only 10 percent of the people who diet just to lose weight are permanently successful, you choose the more powerful combination of cutting caloric intake while increasing the amount of calories you burn every day. You decide that you will evaluate your progress weekly because you know that the above method, if followed properly, will cause you to lose a pound a week. At the end of each week you either reward or punish yourself. The reward must be enticing to you. The reward could be a movie, a book, a record—whatever would be a positive reinforcement of your weight-reducing behavior. The same method can be used to build healthy habits, such as learning to manage your time more effectively and to help you break unhealthy behaviors, although it probably would be best to work on one important behavior change at a time.

Stress can be bad enough when you are dealing with just a few stressors at a time, but you are probably actually facing multiple stressors in your life. This complexity resulting from multiple stressors makes it absolutely necessary for you to approach stress management with the broadest of perspectives, integrating stress-reduction insights and techniques into your life and making the appropriate reinforcing behavioral, psychological, and physical changes. To do any lcss is to be applying bandaids when tourniquets are needed.

One mistake some people make when suffering from distress is to withdraw from the social supports they have in their various relationships. In Chapter 3, we saw that interpersonal relationships can be a source of stress at work, but these relationships can strengthen and encourage you in a time of distress. Of course, not all relationships are of the same quality, and it might be a good idea to assess how well your support network actually helps you. You would not want to be undermined by your own friends, as Job was in the Bible. Learn which people you can turn to for encouragement when you need it, and learn how to mobilize their support. In his studies of Roseto, Pennsylvania, in 1961, John C. Bruhn noted that the incidence of heart disease there was one third the national average and one fourth that of nearby towns. Furthermore, no one under the age of 47 had ever had a heart attack. Traditional community values and closely knit families were highly characteristic of this small mining community, and these were believed to have provided the social support that cushioned the effects of stress upon individuals. However, in 1971 Bruhn found a completely different picture: Life had become more modern, and with the fast-paced living that usually accompanies modernization came a dramatic change in the health of the community—the incidence of heart disease was now equivalent to the national average! Bruhn attributed this significant change largely to the decline in quality or quantity of family and community support which resulted from increasing modernization.

Some of you will want to apply some of the insights and techniques for managing stress to your entire organization, or perhaps at least to your own organizational unit. In the workbook, the sections "Organizational Stressors" and "Three Ways to Increase Productivity in Your Organization" have been provided to encourage and support such an application. (Of course, participation of employees in any such program should be done on a strictly voluntary basis.)

The first step in the process is getting your people to identify key organizational stressors and to assess which ones could be attacked and eliminated—or at least minimized—and which are probably unchangeable. Second, analyze what can be done for each stressor. Third, explore ways in which you may be pushing yourself or others beyond the stress threshold and thus lowering productivity, and find out what can be done to stop it. Fourth, explore ways in which you may be hindering productivity because you aren't putting *enough* stress on others or on yourself.

Managers should encourage their employees to be healthier by using effective stress management strategies. Such encouragement is humanistic and inexpensive (it is inexpensive to encourage people to exercise and to eat properly). In addition, if enough people respond positively to the encouragement, your organization will save money. But in the final analysis, it is up to the individual. You can encourage your people to take action and fight distress but they are the only ones who can do it. You can take responsibility only for yourself. Throughout this book, I have emphasized that stress can be either good or bad for you. You don't want to avoid it all the time; you want to manage it successfully. At times, you need more stress; at other times you need less.

A variety of insights and techniques for managing stress has been presented here because I believe that no single approach is suitable for everybody. I hope that as a result of reading this book and working with the recommended exercises, you will develop your own stress-management strategies tailor-made for your particular situation and personal preferences. Because as I have emphasized throughout this book, *you* ultimately determine how much of an effect stress will have upon you. And *you* ultimately decide how well you will manage it—and whether you can turn stress, that old adversary, into a friend.

Your Personal Stress Management Program: A Workbook

Personal stressors

In the space below, make a list of the things that bother you in your *personal* life. Upon completing the list indicate which stressors can be eliminated or at least minimized and which ones are unlikely to be changeable.

1. ______________________________
2. ______________________________
3. ______________________________
4. ______________________________
5. ______________________________

Organizational stressors

In the space below make a list of the things that bother you in your organization. Upon completing the list, indicate which stressors could be eliminated or at least minimized and which ones are unlikely to be changeable.

1. ______________________________
2. ______________________________
3. ______________________________
4. ______________________________
5. ______________________________

Three ways to raise productivity in your organization*

First: Get the people in your organizational unit to identify what can be done about the stressors in the organization (see your earlier list) that hinder productivity because of the stress impact they have on everyone. Some movement in a positive direction is possible for some of these stressors if a problem-solving approach is taken. Don't spend time on the stressors that can't be changed, once you're sure they can't be.

1. Organizational stressor: ______________________________

   Solution: ______________________________

   ____

2. Organizational stressor: ______________________________

   Solution: ______________________________

   ____

3. Organizational stressor: ______________________________

   Solution: ______________________________

   ____

*Adapted from Jere E. Yates, *Your Own Worst Enemy* (Santa Monica, California Stephen Bosustow Productions, 1978), p. 12. A film on stress with the same title is distributed by Stephen Bosustow Productions.

4. Organizational stressor: ______________________

   Solution: ______________________

   ____

5. Organizational stressor: ______________________

   Solution: ______________________

   ____

Second: Explore ways in which you may be pushing yourself and others beyond the stress threshold and thus lowering productivity.

1. Cause of stress overload: ______________________

   Solution: ______________________

   ____

2. Cause of stress overload: ______________________

   Solution: ______________________

   ____

3. Cause of stress overload: ______________________

   Solution: ______________________

   ____

4. Cause of stress overload: ______________________

   Solution: ______________________

   ____

5. Cause of stress overload: ______________________

   Solution: ______________________

   ____

Third: Explore ways in which you may be hindering productivity because you are not putting *enough* stress on yourself or on others. You may need to motivate people by raising performance expectations.

WHO (INCLUDING YOURSELF) AND WHAT NEEDS MORE STRESS?

1. ______________________________

____

2. ______________________________

____

3. ______________________________

____

4. ______________________________

____

Coping self-statements

Make up coping self-statements to calm you in the following situations. Three or four sentences for each category should be sufficient.

Preparing for a stressful situation ______________________________

____

____

Handling a stressful situation ______________________________

____

____

Coping with the feeling of being overwhelmed ______________________________

____

____

Reinforcing self-statements ______________________________

____

____

Stress reduction through systematic desensitization

Choose a stressful scene that you want to de-stress through systematic desensitization. Briefly describe this scene in space 10, then describe the events immediately leading up to it, in terms of increasing levels of stress, starting with the least stressful scene and proceeding step by step up the hierarchy until you get to the most stressful scene. (See Chapter 5.)

STRESS HIERARCHY

	Scene number	Scene description	Fear thermometer rating
Least stressful scene	0		(0°)
	1		(10°)
	2		(20°)
	3		(30°)
	4		(40°)
	5		(50°)
	6		(60°)
	7		(70°)
	8		(80°)
Most stressful scene	9		(90°)
	10		(100°)

Reprinted from *Asserting Your Self, A Practical Guide for Positive Change* by Sharon Anthony Bower and Gordon H. Bower.

Clarifying your values: an exercise

1. According to your checkbook, what five things do you really value?

2. What would you do if you had one year to live and were guaranteed success in whatever you attempted?

3. What do you regard as your three greatest personal achievements?

4. What do you consider your own greatest personal failure?

5. What three words or qualities would you like to have closely identified with your name, now and after your death?

A physical fitness test

These exercises will give you some indication of your overall state of fitness. If you're under a doctor's care, don't attempt them without your doctor's consent. Stop if you feel overstressed. Do this exercise and then answer the questions with a "yes" or "no."

_____1. When you pinch your waist, while standing, is the skin fold an inch or less?

_____2. Can you hold a deep breath for 45 seconds?

_____3. Is the difference between your chest full of air and your chest not full of air at least 3½ inches if you're a man and 2½ inches if you're a woman?

_____4. Can you do 10 situps?

_____5. Can you do 5 pushups without undue strain?

_____6. Can you step up and down 20 times on a strong chair which is about 15 inches from the floor?

_____7. While sitting on the floor with legs apart and hands clasped behind your head, can you lean forward and touch each elbow to the opposite knee without undue effort?

_____8. Can you do 10 deep knee bends? (Omit this one if you have cartilage problems).

_____9. After running in place for 3 minutes, lifting your feet up at least 4 inches off the floor, is your pulse under 120 beats a minute?

A "no" answer to any of these questions suggests that you are not as physically fit as you should be. If you struggled to complete some of the exercises, you may not be in overall good shape, either.

Source: Adapted from Jack Tresidder (ed.), *Feel Younger, Live Longer,* (Chicago Rand McNally, 1977), pp. 112-113.

Writing your own prescription*

After assessing your own ability to handle stress in your life, be your own doctor and write yourself a prescription indicating specifically what you are going to do to manage stress more effectively.

1. ______________________________

____

____

2. ______________________________

____

____

3. ______________________________

____

____

4. ______________________________

____

____

5. ______________________________

____

____

Signed ______________________

*Adapted from Jere E. Yates, *Your Own Worst Enemy* (Santa Monica, California: Stephen Bosustow Productions, 1978), p. 13.

BIBLIOGRAPHY

"Advice to Businessmen on Health and Retirement," *U.S. News and World Report,* March 7, 1966.

Benson, Herbert. *The Relaxation Response.* New York: William Morrow and Co., 1975.

———, Kotch, Jamie B., Crassweller, Karen D., and Greenwood, Martha M. "Historical and Clinical Considerations of the Relaxation Response," *American Scientist,* July–August, 1977. 441–445.

———, "Your Innate Asset for Combating Stress," *Harvard Business Review,* July–August 1974, 49–60.

Bernstein, Harry. "Work Stress, Strain Claims on the Rise." *Los Angeles Times,* June 8, 1977.

Bloomfield, Harold H., Cain, Michael Peter, Jaffe, Dennis T., and Kory, Robert B. *T.M.: Discovering Inner Energy and Overcoming Stress.* New York: Delacorte Press, 1975.

Bower, Sharon Anthony, and Bower, Gordon H. *Asserting Your Self.* Menlo Park, California: Addison-Wesley, 1976.

Caplan, Robert D.., et. al. *Job Demands and Worker Health: Main Effects and Occupational Differences.* Washington, D.C.: U.S. Department of Health, Education and Welfare, 1975.

Cooper, Gary L., and Marshall, Judi. "Occupational Sources of Stress: A Review of the Literature Relating to Coronary Heart Disease and Mental Ill Health," *Journal of Occupational Psychology,* March 1976.

Cooper, Kenneth H. *Aerobics.* New York: Bantam Books, 1969.

Drucker, Peter. *The Effective Manager.* New York: Harper and Row, 1966.

DuBrin, Andrew J. *Human Relations: A Job Oriented Approach.* Reston, Virginia: Reston Publishing Company, 1978.

Erikson, Erik, H. *Childhood and Society.* New York: W.W. Norton and Co., 1950.

"Formulas for Fitness: How Aerobics Can Help Your Heart—and the Way You Feel," *Readers Digest,* January 1978.

Friedman, Meyer, and Rosenman, Ray H. *Type A Behavior and Your Heart.* Greenwich, Connecticut: Fawcett Publications, 1974.

Fromm, Erich. *The Art of Loving.* New York: Bantam, 1963.

Gallwey, Timothy W. *The Inner Game of Tennis.* New York: Random House, 1974.

Gardner, John W. *Self-Renewal.* New York: Perennial Library, 1971.

Glass, David C. "Stress, Behavior Patterns, and Coronary Disease," *American Scientist,* March–April 1977, pp. 177–187.

Glasser, William. *Reality Therapy.* New York: Harper and Row, 1965.

Goldberg, Philip. *Executive Health.* New York: McGraw-Hill, 1978.

Hamner, Clay W., and Organ, Dennis W. *Organizational Behavior: An Applied Psychological Approach.* Dallas: Business Publications, 1978.

Holmes, Thomas H., and Holmes, T. Stephenson. "How Change Can Make Us Ill," *Stress,* Chicago: Blue Cross Association, 1974.

Jacobson, Edmund. *Progressive Relaxation.* Chicago: University of Chicago Press, 1938.

Janis, Irving. *Victims of Groupthink.* Boston: Houghton Mifflin, 1973.

Johnson, Harry J. *Executive Life-Styles: A Life Extension Institute Report on Alcohol, Sex and Health.* New York: Thomas Y. Crowell Co., 1974.

Kahn, Robert L., and Quinn, Robert P. "Role Stress," *Mental Health and Work Organization,* Chicago: Rand McNally, 1970.

Karlins, Marvin, and Andrews, Lewis M. *Biofeedback: Turning on the Power of Your Mind.* New York: Warner Paperback Library, 1973.

Katz, Daniel, and Kahn, Robert L. *The Social Psychology of Organizations.* New York: John Wiley & Sons, Inc., 1966.

Kelly, Joe. *Organizational Behavior.* New York: Richard D. Irwin, Inc., 1974.

Lamott, Kenneth. *Escape From Stress.* New York: Berkley Medallion Books, 1976.

Laragh, John Henry. "Conquering the Quiet Killer," *Time*, January 13, 1975.

Lecker, Sidney, *The Natural Way to Control Stress*. New York: Grosset and Dunlap, 1978.

Levinson, Harry. *Executive Stress*. New York: Harper and Row, 1966.

Margolis, B. L., Kroes, William H., and Quinn, Robert P., "Job Stress: An Unlisted Occupational Hazard," *Journal of Occupational Medicine*, October 1974, pp. 654–661.

Marrow, Alfred J. (ed.) *The Failure of Success*. New York: AMACOM, 1972.

Marx, Jean L. "Stress: Role in Hypertension Debated," *Science*, December 2, 1977, pp. 905–907.

McQuade, Walter, and Aikman, Ann. *Stress*. New York: Bantam Books, 1975.

Morano, Richard A. "How to Manage Change to Reduce Stress," *Management Review*, November 1977.

Morehouse, Laurence E., and Gross, Leonard. *Total Fitness in 30 Minutes a Week*. New York: Pocket Books, 1976.

Pelletier, Kenneth R. *Mind as Healer, Mind as Slayer*. New York: Delta, 1977.

Peter, Lawrence J., and Hull, Raymond. *The Peter Principle*. New York: William Morrow and Co., 1969.

Peters, Ruanne K., and Benson, Herbert. "Time Out From Tension," *Harvard Business Review*, January–February 1978, pp. 120–124.

Randle, Judy. "Coping with Stress," *Tulsa World*, April 23, 1978.

Robinson, Corinne H. *Fundamentals of Normal Nutrition*. New York: The Macmillan Company, 1973.

Selye, Hans. *Stress Without Distress*. New York: McGraw-Hill Book Company, 1969.

———. *The Stress of Life*. New York: McGraw-Hill Book Company, 1976.

Shaffer, Laurence F., and Shoben, Edward J., Jr. *The Psychology of Adjustment*. New York: Houghton-Mifflin, 1956.

Singer, Jerome E., and Glass, David C. "Making Your World More Liveable," *Stress*. Chicago: Blue Cross, 1974.

Tanner, Ogden, et. al. *Stress*. Alexandria, Virginia: Time-Life Books, 1976.

"The Executive Under Pressure," *Business Week*, May 25, 1974.

Toffler, Alvin. *Future Shock*. New York: Bantam, 1970.

Tresidder, Jack (ed.) *Feel Younger, Live Longer.* Chicago: Rand McNally, 1977.

Weick, Karl E. "The Management of Stress," *MBA Magazine,* October 1975.

Welford, A. T. *Man Under Stress.* New York: John Wiley & Sons, Inc., 1974.

"What You Should Know About Mental Depression," *U.S. News and World Report.* September 9, 1974.

Woolfolk, Robert L., and Richardson, Frank C. *Stress, Sanity, and Survival.* New York: Monarch, 1978.

Yates, Jere E. *Your Own Worst Enemy.* Santa Monica, California: Stephen Bosustow Productions, 1978.

INDEX